Apple Cider VINEGAR

Miracle Health System

with the
BRAGG HEALTHY LIFESTYLE
Vital living at any age

P9-DMD-338

PAUL C. BRAGG, N.D., Ph.D.
LIFE EXTENSION SPECIALIST
and
PATRICIA BRAGG
HEALTH CRUSADER & LIFESTYLE EDUCATOR

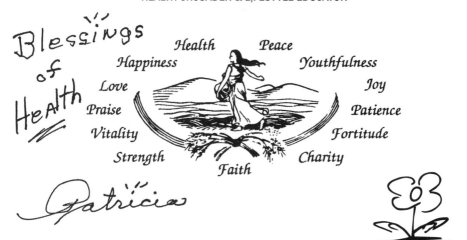

Blessings of Health

Health   Peace

Happiness   Youthfulness

Love   Joy

Praise   Patience

Vitality   Fortitude

Strength   Charity

Faith

Patricia

BECOME
A Health Crusader – for a 100% Healthy World for All!

www.PatriciaBraggBooks.com

Apple Cider
VINEGAR

Miracle Health System

with the
BRAGG HEALTHY LIFESTYLE
Vital living at any age

PAUL C. BRAGG, N.D., Ph.D.
LIFE EXTENSION SPECIALIST
and
PATRICIA BRAGG
HEALTH CRUSADER & LIFESTYLE EDUCATOR

Visit our website:
www.PatriciaBraggBooks.com

Sixtieth Edition MMXXI
ISBN: 978-0-87790-079-5

Library of Congress Cataloging-in-Publication Data on file with publisher

Published in the United States
HEALTH SCIENCE
7127 Hollister Avenue, Suite 25A, Box 249, Santa Barbara, CA 93117
Toll-Free: (833) 408-1122

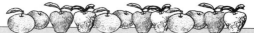

Praises for Apple Cider Vinegar & The Bragg Healthy Lifestyle

For more testimonies see www.PatriciaBraggBooks.com

These are just a few of the thousands of testimonials we receive yearly, praising The Bragg Health Books for the rejuvenation healthy benefits they reap – physically, mentally and spiritually. We look forward to hearing your story, also!

In 1998 I severely broke my left leg and doctors mended it with plates, screws and bolts. I developed staph and pus infections and sores on bottom of my foot. I had constant pain in my foot, ankle and knee. Since then I have had problems walking up and down stairs and kneeling was impossible. Then I started taking organic apple cider vinegar (2 Tbsps 3x a day). Two days after I started, the soreness in my knee disappeared and climbing the stairs is now pain free and all the other problems are gone!!! I never expected all these results, I give full credit to apple cider vinegar. Thank you.
– Duke Jones, Oregonia, OH, Retired Police Officer

Organic apple cider vinegar is great. The vinegar drink has become our life supporting system and we passionately support it and cannot live without it. We thank you for all the many ways we can use apple cider vinegar with the miracle mother enzymes.
– Yasuko and Hiro Hashimoto, former CEO of NEC, Japan

For over 35 years I've followed Bragg Healthy Lifestyle – it teaches you how to take control of your health and build a healthy future.
– Mark Victor Hansen, co-producer, *Chicken Soup For The Soul* Series

When I was a young gymnastics coach at Stanford University, Paul Bragg's words and example inspired me to live a healthy lifestyle. I was twenty-three then; now I'm over sixty, and my health, energy and fitness serves as a living testimonial to Paul C. Bragg's health wisdom, carried on by his dedicated health crusading daughter, Patricia Bragg. Thank you both!
– Dan Millman, author, *The Way of the Peaceful Warrior*
• *www.peacefulwarrior.com*

I lost 102 lbs. with organic apple cider vinegar and The Bragg Healthy Lifestyle and have kept it off for 15 years, staying away from white flour, sugar and other processed foods. – Dee McCaffrey, Chemist & Diet Counselor, Tempe, AZ • *ProcessedFreeAmerica.org*

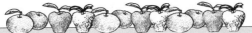

Praises for Apple Cider Vinegar & The Bragg Healthy Lifestyle

Bragg Books were my conversion to the healthy way.
– James F. Balch, M.D., co-author,
Prescription for Nutritional Healing

Paul Bragg saved my life at age 15 when I attended the Bragg Health Crusade in Oakland, California. I thank The Bragg Healthy Lifestyle for my long, healthy, active life spreading health and fitness.
– Jack LaLanne, Bragg follower to 97 • *www.JackLaLanne.com*

Your dad, Dr. Paul Bragg IS the FATHER of the natural health industry and entire natural health movement. Everything that has been done in natural health and physical culture since has been based on the pioneering vision and principles articulated by Dr. Bragg. He gave us all our healthy direction! – Dr. William Wong

As a youth I had a learning disability and was told I would never read, write or communicate normally. At 14 I dropped out of school and at 17 ended up in Hawaii surfing. My road to recovery led me to Paul Bragg who changed my life by giving me one simple affirmation to repeat: "I am a genius and I apply my wisdom." Paul Bragg inspired me to go back to school and get my education and from there miracles happened. I have authored 72 training programs and 40 books and love to crusade around the world thanks to Paul Bragg. – Dr. John Demartini, Dynamic Crusader, Star in *The Secret* • *www.DrDemartini.com*

I love the books and apple cider vinegar! It has made such a difference in my life and to my family. For over a year I was having such terrible skin issues – my skin was peeling like I had a sunburn all the time, I had rosacea and adult acne. Two dermatologists were of no help. No medications, face wash or creams were helping. After meeting you and using ACV as a tonic for my face, it has cleared up to where you would never know I had a problem. I use the ACV as a drink 4 times a day. I lost 6 pounds in 2 weeks following your simple instructions on The Bragg Healthy Lifestyle found in your ACV Book. Thank you for coming into my life when I needed help! Love and Blessings! – Becky, Boca Raton, Florida

Count your blessings, name them one by one; count your many
blessings, see what God hath done. – Johnson Oatman, Jr., songwriter
I give thanks for all the Miracle Blessings I receive daily. – Patricia Bragg

B

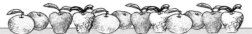

Praises for Apple Cider Vinegar & The Bragg Healthy Lifestyle

I recently bought your *Apple Cider Vinegar* book. I and my whole family use organic apple cider vinegar (with the 'mother') and are committed to following The Bragg Healthy Lifestyle. Thank you. With many Blessings! – Dr. Jan Buscop, South Africa

---

Organic apple cider vinegar is fantastic. Having had stomach problems my entire life, ACV with the "mother" is the only product that has cured my ailment. Thank you so much! – Rebecca Stelling

---

I put daily 2 Tbsps of organic ACV over the feed of my three winning barrel racing horses. It gives them energy, health and beautiful coats. I don't buy equine supplements any more . . . I just get a gallon of organic apple cider vinegar. It works from the inside out. Thank you so much for this GREAT miracle product. – Desiree Dautreuil, Champion Barrel Racer, LaFayette, LA

I have been using organic ACV for 3 months now. I have to say that it has literally changed my life and my body. I started taking ACV just to build up my immune system and WOW did it bring some extra-ordinary changes besides keeping me from getting ill. My results from using ACV with the "mother" – I lost 20 lbs. and energy levels went through the roof! After a heavy work out, I hardly get sore. Also I was plagued by yeast infections. Happy they are now gone! Bowel movements are like clockwork. ACV is a wonderful product and I fully and truly recommend it. It really has changed my life! – Linda W., Michigan

---

Thanks to you and your wonderful father for your guidance and teaching over the years. What a great gift you and your father have provided for us all through your Bragg Health Books. Your *Miracle of Fasting* and *Apple Cider Vinegar* books have improved my life immensely. I've lost 30 lbs. and feel years younger. At 67 youthful years, I give thanks for the great benefits of health I enjoy because of the work you and your father have so generously dedicated your lives too!! Wishing you every blessing under the Sun. – Captain Wes Herman (retired) Santa Barbara County Fire Dept.

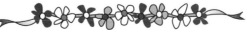

Change your mind – change to a healthy lifestyle and your life and body will sparkle with health and joy! – Patricia Bragg, Lifestyle Educator

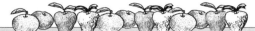

Praises for Apple Cider Vinegar & The Bragg Healthy Lifestyle

I had an issue with gallstones and was told by my doctor that an operation was the only way to get rid of them. A friend gave me page 23 of the *Bragg Apple Cider Vinegar* book and I tried the flush. It helped and 2 years later I have not had any pains and have not needed the operation! I bought a copy of the book, and have been using the ACV ever since. It's a great product. – Nicole, Jamaica

My parents, 91 and 86 are keeping youthful and enjoying vinegar drinks, it helps with so many things! We appreciate your teachings more than you know!! – Barbara Magiley, San Antonio, TX

Hello, I have always had PMS or cramps. But since taking organic apple cider vinegar drink I am thankful it helped resolve the problem and irritability that used to ruin my day.
– Paula Bowen, Wisconsin

I have an amazing story to tell you about organic apple cider vinegar. I've been struggling with high cholesterol for 6 years now, and couldn't seem to get it down by exercising and watching what I ate. Doctors were concerned, so my mom told me to try organic apple cider vinegar. I did it 3 months straight faithfully – a tablespoon twice a day. Just went for my blood test, and can't believe it! I dropped 78 points in just 3 months, it's amazing! My doctors are asking me, "what's the secret?" They can't believe it either. I just thought I'd let you know that ACV really does work. Thank you so much. – Jamie, Massachusetts

I would like to share with you what organic ACV has done for me. I had a blood test to check my cholesterol. I was shocked at the numbers – 275 total (50 HDL and 193 LDL). After using organic apple cider vinegar for 3 months, it helped me maintain normal cholesterol levels. My doctor was shocked; he asked me how and I said organic apple cider vinegar. No medication for me. Thanks for a healthy way of life. I use one gallon purified water mixed with 1/2 bottle (8 oz.) organic ACV with raw honey. One glass in the morning and one glass in the evening. I thank God and His blessings for you and your people. Please share this with others. – Barbara Darnell, Ohio

Be your own Health Captain and do what needs to be done for your health!

D

Praises for Apple Cider Vinegar & The Bragg Healthy Lifestyle

I have suffered with an irritable bowel, colitis, spastic colon, constipation and unnatural, painful gas for years. I have been on all kinds of medicine. Nothing seemed to work, until I started taking the organic apple cider vinegar. Wow! My problem is gone! Why didn't somebody tell me about this sooner? I now have my life back and can socialize again. – Fran Covert, Colorado

I had the opportunity to sit next to Patricia on a flight from Dallas to L.A. Her honesty about my weight and health really inspired me to make a life change. One year later, I am 85 lbs. lighter and heart rate cut almost in half. Patricia you helped save my life! – Mike Ableman, Texas

In 1975 I was diagnosed with coronary heart disease. I started following the Free Bragg Exercise Classes and Lectures at Fort DeRussy in Waikiki, 6 times a week and I now feel young again thanks to The Bragg Healthy Lifestyle. In 1932 my father had severe hip arthritis and was hardly able to walk. He followed Paul Bragg's Healthy Lifestyle too with vinegar drink and was cured of his arthritis. – Helen, R.N., Hawaii

As the world's foremost authority on human memory performance, I tell all my students that one cannot have optimum memory without taking organic apple cider vinegar. I've been taking ACV all my life. To have a healthy memory you need a healthy brain and to have a healthy brain you need organic ACV. – David, the "Memory Man", California

Our great-grandmother will turn 100 in two weeks. She still kayaks, gardens, and shovels her own snow covered driveway. For over 80 years, she had one recipe for life: 2 Tbsps organic ACV and 1 tsp of honey mixed into water. This is the secret, she says, to a life worth living. Five generations of our family will celebrate her 100th birthday with Vinegar Drinks! – The Alvina Sharp Family, Chanhassen, Minnesota

Obey the Laws of Mother Nature and God and you will see results you now scarcely dare to dream! Miracles will happen! – Patricia Bragg

Pray for wisdom in your daily living – for more faith and patience with yourself and others before you pray for just things. – Patricia Bragg

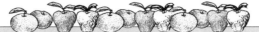

Praises for Apple Cider Vinegar & The Bragg Healthy Lifestyle

How did I beat cancer, obesity, diabetes, strep, three herniated disks and excruciating pain? The answer was changing to The Bragg Healthy Lifestyle and having the amazing organic apple cider vinegar drink daily. It changed my life and I also lost 70 lbs! I received a new life and that is just the beginning because my manhood returned that was lost to diabetes – now that's exciting! On my trip to Honolulu I visited the famous free Bragg Exercise Class at Waikiki Beach. I became so regenerated with a wonderful new viewpoint towards living The Bragg Healthy Lifestyle that I now live in Hawaii. I'm invigorated with new energy for life and living! My new purpose for living is to help others reclaim their health rights! I want the world to join The Health Crusade. I am so thankful to Paul and Patricia for being my inspiration. – Len, Hawaii

---

Thanks to the ageless Bragg Health Books, they were our introduction to healthy living. We are very grateful to you and your father. – Marilyn Diamond, Co-Author, "Fit For Life" Best Seller – 40 weeks

---

Thank you Paul and Patricia Bragg for my simple, easy to follow Healthy Lifestyle. You make my days healthy!
– Clint Eastwood, Academy Award Winning Film Producer, Director, Actor and Bragg follower for over 60 years

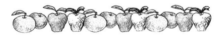

See more ACV & Bragg Health Teaching Praises on pages 127-128

We get letters daily at our Santa Barbara headquarters. We would love to receive a testimonial letter from you on any blessings, healings and changes you experienced after following The Bragg Healthy Lifestyle and this book. It's all within your grasp to be in top health. By following this book, you can reap more Super Health and a happy, longer vital life! It's never too late to begin. Studies show amazing results that were obtained with people in their 80's and 90's (pages 83-86). Receive miracles with healthy nutrition, fasting and exercise! Don't wait – start now!

Daily our prayers & love go out to you, your heart, mind & soul with love.

Patricia Bragg

3 John 2

F | *Miracles can happen every day through guidance and prayer! – Patricia Bragg*

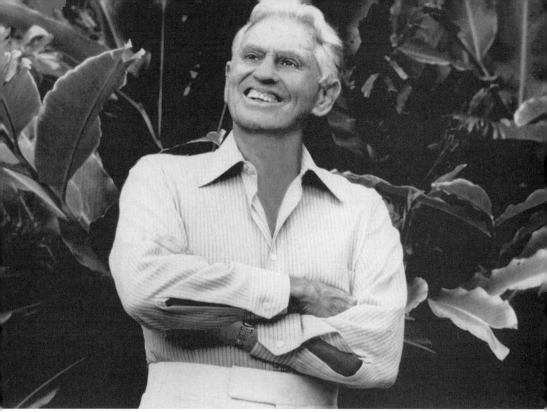

PAUL C. BRAGG, N.D., Ph.D.
World's Leading Healthy Lifestyle Authority

Paul C. Bragg's daughter Patricia and their wonderful, healthy members of the Bragg *Longer Life, Health and Happiness Club* exercised daily on the beautiful Fort DeRussy lawn, at famous Waikiki Beach in Honolulu, Hawaii. On Saturday there were often health lectures on how to live a long, healthy life! The group averaged 50 to 75 per day, depending on the season. From December to March it can go up to 125. Its dedicated leaders carried on the class for over 43 years. Thousands visited the club from around the world and carried the Bragg Health and Fitness Crusade to friends and relatives back home.

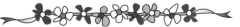

Your body is a non-stop living system, in constant motion 24 hours daily, cleaning, repairing, healing and growing. – Patricia Bragg

To maintain good health, normal weight and increase the good life of radiant health, joy and happiness, the body must be exercised properly (stretching, walking, jogging, biking, swimming, deep breathing, good posture) and nourished with healthy foods. – Paul C. Bragg, N.D., Ph.D.

iii

❀ Cautionary Note and Disclaimer ❀

The information provided here is for educational purposes only. Any decision on your part to read, listen and use this information is your personal choice. The information in this book is not meant to be used to diagnose, prescribe or treat any illness. Please discuss any changes you wish to make to your medical treatment with a qualified, licensed health care provider.

If you are taking medication to control your blood sugar or blood pressure, you may need to reduce the dosage if you significantly restrict your carbohydrate intake. This is best done under the care and supervision of an experienced and qualified licensed health care provider. Anyone who has any other serious illness such as cardiovascular disease, cancer, kidney or liver disease needs to exercise caution if making dietary changes. You should consult your physician for guidance. If you are pregnant or lactating, you should not overly restrict protein or fat intake. Also, young children and teens have much more demanding nutrient needs and should NOT have their protein or fat intake overly restricted.

The information presented in this book is in no way intended as medical advice or a substitute for medical counseling. It is intended only to provide the opinions and ideas of the authors. It is sold with the understanding that the authors are not engaged in rendering medical, health or any other kind of professional services in this book. The reader should consult his or her medical doctor, or any other competent professional, before adopting any of the suggestions in this book, or drawing inferences from it.

The authors disclaim any responsibility for any liability, loss or risk, personal or otherwise, which is incurred as a consequence, directly or indirectly, of the use and application of the contents of this book.

Please consult your physician before beginning this program, and use all of the information the authors suggest in conjunction with the guidance and care of your physician. Your physician should be aware of all medical conditions that you may have, as well as medications and supplements you are taking.

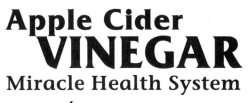

Apple Cider VINEGAR
Miracle Health System

In 400 B.C., Hippocrates, the Father of Medicine, treated his patients with amazing raw Apple Cider Vinegar because he recognized its powerful cleansing and healing qualities. It's a naturally occurring antibiotic and antiseptic that fights germs, viruses, bacteria, even mold.

 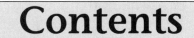 **Contents**

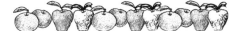

 "Who satisfieth thy mouth with good things, so that thy youth is renewed like the eagle's." – Psalms 103:5

Check out this web for amazing ways to use Bragg Apple Cider Vinegar:
DoctorOz.com/article/101-clever-ways-use-apple-cider-vinegar

v

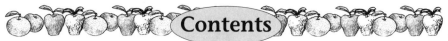

Contents

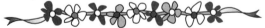

When you sell a man a book you don't just sell him paper, ink and glue, you sell him a whole new life! There's heaven and earth in a real book. The real purpose of books is to inspire the mind to do its own thinking!
– Christopher Morley, Honored American Journalist and Poet

You can change and improve the quality of your health by detoxifying and cleansing your body with your Bragg Healthy Lifestyle. Start today!

The more natural food you eat, the more you'll enjoy radiant health and be able to promote the higher life of love and brotherhood.
– Patricia Bragg

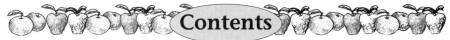

Contents

 Bragg Healthy Lifestyle Plan

- *Read, plan, plot, and follow through for supreme health and longevity.*
- *Underline, highlight or dog-ear pages as you read important passages.*
- *Organizing your lifestyle helps you identify what's important in your life.*
- *Be faithful to your health goals everyday for a healthy, long, happy life.*
- *Where space allows we have included "words of wisdom" from great minds to motivate and inspire you! Please share your favorite sayings with us.*
- *Write us about your successes following The Bragg Healthy Lifestyle.*

Where there is great love, there are always miracles. – Willa Cather

Check out this video on beneficial effects of Apple Cider Vinegar: vimeo.com/155145288. More info on this study on pages 16-17.

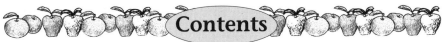

Contents

We must always improve, renew, rejuvenate ourselves; otherwise, we harden. – Johann Wolfgang von Goethe

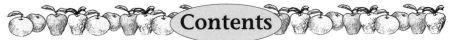

Contents

---

*Listen to your body carefully, you will hear it clearly when you sit
in silence and observe your breath. – Peeyush Bhargava, M.D.*

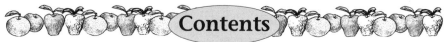

Contents

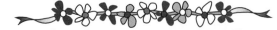

Ten Tips for Good Health

- *Respect and protect your body as the highest manifestation of your life.*
- *Abstain from unnatural, devitalized foods and stimulating beverages.*
- *Nourish your body with only natural unprocessed, live foods.*
- *Extend your years in health for loving, sharing and charitable service.*
- *Regenerate your body by the right balance of activity and rest.*
- *Purify your cells, tissue and blood with healthy organic foods, and with pure water, clean air and gentle sunshine.*
- *Abstain from all food when out of sorts in mind or body.*
- *Keep thoughts, words and emotions pure, calm, loving and uplifting.*
- *Increase your knowledge of Mother Nature's Laws, follow them, and enjoy the fruits of your life's labor.*
- *Lift up yourself, friends and family by loyal obedience to Mother Nature's and God's Healthy, Natural Laws of Living.*

"Love all, trust a few, do wrong to none." – William Shakespeare

Apple Cider Vinegar Miracle Health System

 **The Powerful Health Qualities of Natural Apple Cider Vinegar**

Research worldwide supports and commends what Hippocrates (the father of medicine) found and treated his patients with in 400 B.C. He discovered that natural, undistilled apple cider vinegar (or ACV)***** is a powerful cleansing and healing elixir – a naturally occurring antibiotic and antiseptic that fights germs, bacteria, mold and viruses – for a healthier, stronger, longer life!

Versatility of ACV as a powerful body cleansing agent and weight reduction agent is legendary. It's traced to Egyptian urns back to 3000 B.C. The Babylonians used it as a condiment and preservative, while Julius Caesar's army used ACV tonic to stay healthy and fight off disease. The Greeks and Romans kept vinegar vessels for healing and flavoring. It was used in Biblical times as an antiseptic and a healing agent and is mentioned in the Bible. In Paris in the Middle Ages it was sold from barrels by street vendors as a body deodorant, healing tonic and delicious vinegar drink to help keep the body healthy and ageless.

Even Christopher Columbus on his voyage to discover America in 1492 had vinegar barrels for prevention of scurvy as did Captain James Cook on his ships to the South Seas. It helped disinfect and heal the U.S. Civil War soldiers wounds. For centuries in Japan, the feared Samurai warriors drank it for power. The Chinese call vinegar a "friend" because they have used it for centuries to process herbal medicines. ACV has been used for thousands of years not only for health reasons, but as a cleansing agent to remove bacteria, germs, mold, odors, even stains and spots.

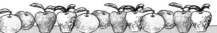

*The best vinegar is organic, raw, unfiltered, unpasteurized Apple Cider Vinegar with the miracle "Mother Enzyme."

ACV – Mother Nature's Perfect Miracle Food

Natural (undistilled) organic, raw ACV can be called one of Mother Nature's most perfect foods, the world's first natural medicine. It is made from fresh, crushed apples which are then allowed to mature naturally in wooden barrels to "boost" the natural fermentation. Natural ACV is a rich, light golden color and held to light you might see tiny formation of "cobweb-like" substances we call the miracle "mother." Usually some "mother enzyme" settles at the bottom of the bottle as it ages. It never needs refrigeration! You can also save some "mother" and transfer it to other natural vinegars. When you smell natural ACV, often there is a pungent odor and sometimes it can pucker your mouth and smart your eyes – these are natural, good signs.

ACV Has Proven Powerful Health Qualities*

The healthy miracle nutrients that live in the "mother" substance of organic, unfiltered, fully ripened ACV have proven powerful health benefits! ACV helps extract calcium from fruits and vegetables, helping to maintain strong bones. ACV is also loaded with potassium. Studies have shown potassium helps prevent hair loss, brittle teeth and nails, sinusitis, runny nose, toxic waste in the body, plus stunted growth! The beta-carotene in ACV helps fight harmful free radicals and breaks down unwanted fat to aid in weight management. ACV contains malic acid, which relieves fungal and bacterial infections, as well as helps dissolve the uric acid deposits that form around your joints. (pages 26-27)

Sadly, commercial producers distill their vinegar to meet consumer demand that vinegar be clear. In distilling, the vinegar is turned to steam by heating.

* *Most of the scientific sourcing for the health statements about apple cider vinegar found in this book can be located in the multiple research studies hosted on the National Institutes of Health website, (nih.gov). The National Institutes of Health is part of the US Department of Health & Human Services. These scientific studies were conducted in the United States and in many different countries around the world.*

Therefore it destroys the powerful "mother enzymes" and distills out life-giving minerals such as potassium, phosphorus, natural organic sodium, magnesium, sulphur, iron, copper, natural organic fluorine, silicon, trace minerals, essential amino acids and many other powerful nutrients including pectin, a fiber that helps reduce bad cholesterol and helps to regulate blood pressure. Distilling also destroys the natural malic and tartaric acids which are important in fighting body toxins and inhibiting unfriendly bacteria.

Apples Are Rich in Potassium and Enzymes

"An apple a day keeps the doctor away" is a familiar wise saying to millions. **The apple is one of Mother Nature's great health-giving foods.** Apples contain enzymes, boron, iron, minerals, trace minerals, pectin-soluble fiber and are a good source of potassium, which is to the soft body tissues as calcium is to the bones and harder tissues. Potassium is the mineral of youthfulness; it's the "artery softener," helping keep arteries of the body flexible and resilient. It's a fighter of dangerous bacteria, viruses and helps dissolve fat. Yes, when you say, "An apple a day keeps the doctor away," this is good, down-to-earth old-fashioned folk medicine for vibrant, life-long health! Since the Garden of Eden the apple has played a vital part in our destiny. People have been eating apples for thousands of years. Apple eaters have a certain healthfulness that non-apple eaters are missing out on.

3

Apples are delicious fruits that most people enjoy eating, but we look upon the organic apple as more than something good to eat. Potassium is the key mineral in the constellation of minerals; it's so important to every living thing that without it there would be no life! Most humans are potassium deficient (page 5) and it reflects in their cell tissues and throughout their entire body. Look around you. How many people do you see that have the super apple glow of health?

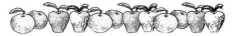

ACV is healthy and nutritious for all ages – including pregnant women.

Millions Suffer From Potassium Deficiency

Millions of people living in today's civilization and eating commercialized, processed foods have a potassium deficiency. The skin and muscle tone are bad. The flesh does not cling firmly to the body's bony framework. Lines and wrinkles fill the face and neck. The hair is brittle.

One sign is flabby, excess skin hanging over the eyes. If the potassium deficiency continues, the prolapsing eyelids progress. Soon, people are looking out of slits instead of wide-open eyes. Thousands have turned to eyelid surgery to correct droopy eyelids, also called hooded eyelids, that roll down and rest on their eyelashes causing eyestrain, headaches, etc. If an eye doctor suggests corrective surgery for this, the insurance company usually honors the claim. It's an in/out local procedure. It's wise to have a board certified eye surgeon. People wrongly blame their age for their droopy eyelids, skin changes and lack of muscle tone.

But the truth is . . . you must have potassium to build and maintain youthful, healthy tissues! If you don't get the required amount of potassium daily, you soon acquire a tired look and feel. This premature ageing is usually due to a potassium deficiency and unhealthy living!

It is the same in your flower and vegetable garden. Potassium is necessary for the health production of the substances that give rigidity to plant stems and increase their resistance to the many diseases that attack plants. Potassium is also the powerful element that changes seeds into plants and beautiful flowers by progressive development. If plants become deficient in potassium, they stop their growth. If the potassium deficiency is not corrected, the plant slowly starts to wither, turns yellow and dies! The same is true of animals and humans with a potassium deficiency: there is a slow degeneration leading to death of the cells, then death of life.

Through his contact with country medicine practiced for 300 years in Vermont, our friend, Dr. D.C. Jarvis stated potassium in its natural combination with other trace minerals is so essential to the metabolic process in every form of life on Earth, that without it there would be no life! Taking ACV promotes a potassium-rich blood chemistry to help keep body tissues soft, pliable and helps prevent hardening of the arteries.

Some Body Signs of Potassium Deficiency

- Bone and muscle aches and pains, especially lower back.

- The body feels heavy, tired and it's an effort to move.

- Shooting pains when straightening up after leaning over.

- Dizziness upon straightening up after leaning over.

- Morning dull headaches upon arising and when stressed.

- Dull, faded-looking hair that lacks sheen and luster.

- The scalp is itchy and dry. Dandruff, premature hair thinning or balding may occur.

- The hair is unmanageable, mats, often looks straw-like, and is sometimes extremely dry and other times oily.

- The eyes itch, feel sore and uncomfortable and appear bloodshot and watery. Also, eyelids may be granulated with white matter collecting in the corners.

- The eyes tire easily and will not focus as they should.

- You tire physically and mentally with the slightest effort.

- Loss of mental alertness and onset of confusion, making decisions difficult. The memory fails, making you forget familiar names and places you should easily remember.

- You become easily irritable and impatient with family, friends and loved ones and even with your business and social acquaintances at times.

- You feel nervous, depressed, in a mental fog, and have difficulty getting things done due to mental and muscle fatigue. Sadly, even the slightest effort can leave you exhausted, upset and sometimes even trembling.

- At times, your hands and feet get chilled, even in warm weather, which is a strong sign of potassium deficiency.

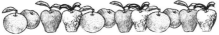

Potassium deficiency is a proven contributing cause of many illnesses, including: arthritis, kidney stones, diabetes, adrenal insufficiency, Celiac Disease, stroke, high blood pressure, coronary artery disease, lupus, hypothyroidism, irritable bowel syndrome, Alzheimer's, Multiple Sclerosis, atrial fibrillation, Crohn's Disease and atherosclerosis.
– Linda Page, N.D., Ph.D., author of "Healthy Healing"

Refined Foods and Flours Remove Vital Potassium which Causes Poor Health!

Robbed grains: The miller refines and processes our grains to get white flour that will keep for years . . . that becomes the staff of death! Even bugs have more sense – they won't eat it because it has been robbed of its potassium and vital life-giving nutritional qualities!

Shocking loss of potassium and nutrients in making white flour: In milling wheat, the miller refines out 25 important food elements, including vital amino acids, vitamin E, bran, the rich B-complex vitamins and potassium. Cows fed refined grain, with the potassium milled out and de-germed, die early of heart failure.

The more vital potassium is refined out of foods, the sicker Americans get: People waste money, time, and energy and suffer the loss of health by being sick. **The #1 health plan should be to teach Americans how to live a healthy lifestyle that maintains health by correct eating and living habits!** Healthy nutrition will create bones that last a lifetime, cells that resist disease and arteries that stay healthy, cholesterol-free and unclogged!

6

Potassium Deficiency Can Stunt Growth and Shorten Lifespan

We have enjoyed making over 10 scientific health expeditions throughout the world, studying the health, the longevity and growth of various races of people. We found areas where the topsoil was deficient in potassium and the people living off foods grown from this potassium-deficient soil were prone to be stunted in growth and have a shorter lifespan. The pygmies of Africa are stunted and short-lived. The same is true of the Arctic Eskimos. In their daily diet, they just do not get the required amount of potassium and other minerals that are so important to growth, health and long life.

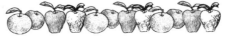

Potassium is the key mineral in the constellation of minerals; it's so important to every living thing that without it there would be no life. Organic Raw Apple Cider Vinegar is a rich source of potassium.

Potassium Deficiency Produces Senility

Throughout the world, there are millions of senile, prematurely old people. Many don't know their own names, nor can they recognize their family or closest friends. They are just barely existing. It might seem that they have degenerated so much that it's almost a hopeless task to try to save them, but please try! We feel they can be restored to useful lives if the toxic poisons are flushed from their bodies and their nutritional deficiencies (vitamins, potassium and niacin) are corrected!

Miracle Potassium Cleans Your Arteries

Years ago, we selected four senile people we felt could be helped. We put them on The Bragg Healthy Lifestyle with the ACV drink and healthy foods rich in potassium. Out of the four, we were able to save three of them. All three left the convalescent home where they had been confined and became healthy, happy and self-sufficient! Two of them made remarkable recoveries. One went back to contracting and building at 80, and the other in his mid 80s resumed his accounting career!

Most senile people suffer from a clogged arterial system. Potassium is to the soft tissues of the body as calcium is to the hard structures. The potassium goes into the clogged, caked arteries and cleans out the rust and dirt just like vinegar water removes grime from windows (page 123). One can't think clearly if arteries are heavily clogged with cholesterol and toxic poisons.

Potassium might be called the great detergent of the arteries. Potassium slows down hardening and clogging processes that cause deadly harm to the whole cardiovascular system. Organic, raw ACV contains miraculous potassium that also makes flesh of farm animals healthier and more tender. There is very little doubt, in animal and man, that the main function of potassium is to keep tissues healthy, soft and pliable, which helps to prevent heart attacks and strokes!

Potassium is necessary for pH balance of your body and for normal blood pressure regulation. Potassium is also needed for muscle growth, nervous system and brain function. It's found in many different fruits and veggies.

Paul's Father Used ACV for Chronic Fatigue

My father was a splendid farmer and many times I would watch him add ACV to the feed and water of ailing animals (cattle, horses, sheep, dogs, cats, and birds) and it acted like magic. ACV seemed to possess a miracle ingredient that helped restore health to the animals. See page 125 for more tips on healthy pets.

The nearest doctor was 32 miles from our home. If a doctor was needed, he had to come by horse and buggy over miles of rough, dirt roads. So, at our home we developed simple self-health remedies and apple cider vinegar played an important health role.

I remember when my father would put in long hours at the farm during the harvest period. He was up long before daybreak and didn't retire until late at night. I would watch him come into the kitchen, put 2 heaping tsps. of honey in a glass, add 2 tsps. of raw apple cider vinegar, fill the glass with water and then sip it slowly.

 I would ask, "Father, why do you drink apple cider vinegar, honey and water?" Father would reply, "Son, farm work is long, hard work. It can produce extreme body fatigue. Whatever is in this apple cider vinegar and honey drink relieves me of that chronic fatigue."

Father was definitely correct. There was an ingredient in that drink that renewed his vitality and relieved him of the chronic fatigue and stiffness. That ingredient was potassium, along with the powerful enzymes, minerals and trace elements that are in organic, raw apple cider vinegar.

Most people today, when they work hard, often turn to all kinds of dangerous, toxic stimulants to relieve their chronic fatigue: alcohol, tea, coffee, cola drinks and pep pills and other dangerous, unhealthy addictive drugs.

My father's good advice fell on youthful ears. It was some years later that I realized that my father was a smart man in using raw honey and raw apple cider vinegar, rich in potassium, to combat chronic fatigue.

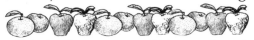

Man is the sole and absolute master of his own fate forever. What he has sown in times of his ignorance, he must inevitably reap; when he attains enlightenment, it is for him to sow what he chooses and reap accordingly. – Geraldine Coster, author, "Yoga and Western Psychology"

Dr. Carrel's Eternal Life Study Successful

Nobel Scientist Dr. Alexis Carrel of the Rockefeller Institute in New York in 1912 kept the cells of an embryo chicken heart alive and healthy for over 35 years by daily monitoring its complete nutrition, cleansing and elimination. A chicken's lifespan averages 7 years!

Apple cider vinegar was given to the chicken embryo daily for its full quota of potassium. Dr. Carrel definitively proved to the entire world that the body has a seed of eternal life! He could have continued this experiment indefinitely to give the embryo immortality, but felt 35 years proved the point that man kills himself by his wrong habits of overeating and living an unhealthy lifestyle! This study showed us the importance of nutrition, cleansing and how apple cider vinegar is vital to life, health and longevity! Web:

nobel prize.org/nobel_prizes/medicine/
laureates/1912/carrel-bio.html

More Health Benefits of Raw, Organic ACV

One of the greatest benefits of ACV is that it detoxifies both the bloodstream and various organs of the body. ACV acts as a purifier, breaking down fatty mucous and phlegm. It also prevents your urine from becoming excessively alkaline, assisting your vital organs – kidneys, bladder and liver. ACV also helps promote healthy blood flow to your heart, brain and your entire body.

Other incredible benefits of ACV are the relief of constipation, headaches, arthritis, indigestion, diarrhea, eczema, sore eyes, chronic fatigue, mild food poisoning, as well as high blood pressure and heartburn symptoms.

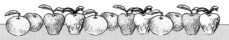

Raw honey has miraculous nutrients (vitamins, potassium and enzymes). It's a natural occurring antibiotic and antiseptic. Ancient Egyptian medicine touted honey as essential natural cure-all, listing 500 honey remedies. Hippocrates, prescribed honey as it fights bacteria, ulcers, infection, combats inflammation, reduces pain, improves circulation, stimulates regrowth of tissue, makes healing faster and reduces scarring. ACV & honey together are nature's perfect cure!
– benefits-of-honey.com

Animals and pets can greatly benefit taking apple cider vinegar: from cats and dogs to parrots, chickens, horses, cows, zebras. It deters insects such as fleas, ticks and mosquitoes; relieves skin and ear problems; prevents intestinal upsets; reduces excess weight; promotes a healthy shiny coat; eliminates cat urine odor and even can take away the smell of stinky skunks!

People ask us about the merits and benefits of ACV. See inside front cover for list of miracles it can perform and has for centuries. **Please read testimonies on pages:** A-F, 15, 23, 26, 27, 32, 38, 41, 75, 81, 86, 127-137.

ACV Kills Germs, Viruses, Mold and Bacteria

Recent studies show a straight 5% solution of vinegar kills 99% of bacteria, 82% of common mold and 80% of germs and viruses. It's a great germ and virus fighter in homes, kitchens, baths and hospitals and labs. Some mix it with water to wash windows, as it removes sludge and keeps them sparkling clean, as apple cider vinegar does for the body. Apple cider vinegar has hundreds of uses and its versatility is legendary as a powerful household cleaner, deodorizing agent and disinfectant, and it's free of dangerous chemicals. (Use white vinegar for cleaning, see pages 121 to 125.)

Why Has Natural Apple Cider Vinegar Disappeared from Grocers' Shelves?

The blame for the disappearance of natural raw apple cider vinegar from supermarkets lies on the shoulders of the general public, as well as the producers of vinegar. Most people buy food with their eyes, not thinking of good nutrition. Vinegar producers failed to enlighten

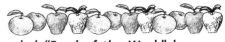

Vinegar was awarded "Food of the Week" because of its healing and cleansing properties and for its anti-cancer elements. – Vinegar Institute

Paul C. Bragg talks about vinegar miracles on family farm in youth. "I was raised on a large farm and we grew many varieties of apples. I was a great apple eater. My father made natural apple cider vinegar and stored it in wooden barrels. On our table daily we used this natural apple cider vinegar and vinegar drinks and our family thrived and loved it."

the public on what powerful health qualities are locked within natural ACV. Why? Because they didn't know the health values of natural, raw, organic, unfiltered, cloudy (to some, less attractive-looking) ACV with the "mother." They produced pasteurized, refined, distilled vinegars because the public preferred it. Filling current supply and demand tragically removed the priceless miraculous "mother" health benefits.

Powerful Health Qualities They Removed

You cannot completely blame the producers of vinegar. They are not nutritionists, nor are they biochemists. Their business is to give the customers what they want. Most people purchase vinegar for flavoring, also for pickling and marinating their foods. Some women use it to rinse their hair after shampooing, as it leaves the hair squeaky clean, softer and much easier to manage.

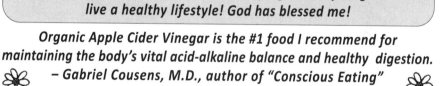

Paul C. Bragg says . . . "Life is thrilling when you can help others!" I founded the Health Movement and originated, named and started the first Health Food Store. Then, through Bragg Health Crusades, I inspired hundreds of Bragg students to open the first Health Food Stores in their areas across America and then worldwide! It's thrilling and rewarding to live a life of service helping and inspiring others to live a healthy lifestyle! God has blessed me!

Organic Apple Cider Vinegar is the #1 food I recommend for maintaining the body's vital acid-alkaline balance and healthy digestion.
– Gabriel Cousens, M.D., author of "Conscious Eating"

There is no wealth greater than the health of the body. – The Bible

Hippocrates, the Father of Medicine, in 400 B.C. treated his patients with amazing raw Apple Cider Vinegar because he recognized its powerful cleansing and healing qualities. It is a naturally occurring antibiotic and antiseptic that fights germs and bacteria in the body.

Every man is the builder of a temple called his body . . . We are all sculptors and painters and our material is our own flesh and blood and bones. Any nobleness begins at once to refine a man's features, and any meanness or sensuality to imbrute them. – Henry David Thoreau

The strongest principle of growth lies in the human choice. – George Eliot

Commercial Vinegars are Real Tragedies

Then came the real tragedy: a food chemist produced an imitation vinegar from coal tar! It looked clean, white and tasted like vinegar. Today it's the most popular vinegar in supermarkets. It's cheaper than malt vinegar or distilled vinegar. Most people buy these worthless vinegars. There's nothing good about commercial vinegars, except they look clean and taste like vinegar. They have no health value! They don't contain the health values of organic, raw ACV with the 'mother.' Sad fact: millions worldwide never get the health benefits of this natural organic apple cider vinegar as wise Doctor Hippocrates used in 400 B.C. Many people have some preconceived idea that apple cider vinegar is harmful to the body. Instead it's the distilled, pasteurized, filtered, white, malt and synthetic, dead vinegars that must be avoided for human consumption!

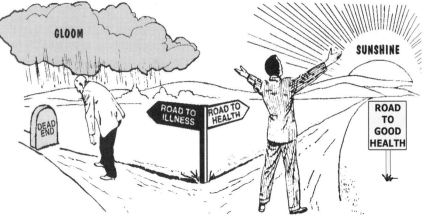

NEGATIVE ⇦ OR ⇨ POSITIVE
The choice of which road to take is up to you.

You alone decide whether to reach a dead end or live a healthy lifestyle for a long, healthy, happy, fulfilled life. – Paul C. Bragg

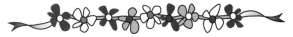

A healthy diet, along with Apple Cider Vinegar and The Bragg Healthy Lifestyle will bring remarkable results. – "Woman's World Magazine"

Slash Artery Plaque with ACV: A Japanese Corporate News Network (JCNN) study found that regular intake of ACV (3 tsps. or more per day) can naturally and significantly reduce the level of cholesterol plaque in blood.

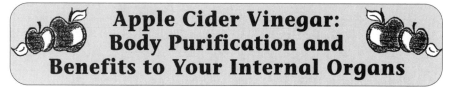

Apple Cider Vinegar: Body Purification and Benefits to Your Internal Organs

Purify Your Cells by Ridding The Body of Dangerous Toxic Wastes

Toxic poisons are the cause of most troubles in the human body. Most people do not have sufficient vital force to supply the eliminative organs with the strength to remove normal waste from the body. The toxins remain and lodge in the joints and organs of the body. We have a name for each symptom that gives us pain and trouble. Certain toxic wastes that are harmful to the whole body are rendered harmless by a miraculous substance in organic, raw ACV with the powerful 'mother enzyme.' Scientists call this protective action *acetolysis*.

Apple Cider Vinegar for Body Purification

It's time for life changes when you feel badly and don't seem to have the Human Go Power and Vital Force to do the things in life that are necessary! It's time to flush out the energy depleting, problem causing toxic wastes that are clogging your machinery and organs of elimination! Waste products broken down by this ACV process are flushed out. **Remember, your important organs of elimination are the bowel, lungs, skin and kidneys. They are your faithful servants!** They work hard 24 hours a day to detox and flush out toxic wastes. Many times these eliminative organs need help and that is when the ACV drink comes to their aid!

Follow ACV daily program. In addition, add 1 tsp. ACV to 6 ounces of salt-free tomato or fresh vegetable juice (carrot and greens) and drink between meals, daily. Do a cleansing fast one day weekly (pages 105-110) and faithfully follow *The Bragg Healthy Lifestyle*, which is explained throughout the book in full, simple details.

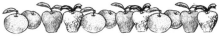

With fasting the quick, safe and effective elimination of dead cells stimulates the building and growth of new healthy cells. – Paul C. Bragg, N.D., Ph.D.

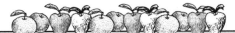

Eat Plenty of Raw Cabbage
– A Miracle Cleanser and Healer

Cabbage (raw) has amazing properties. It stimulates the immune system, kills bacteria and viruses, heals ulcers, and according to Dr. James Balch in "Prescription for Cooking and Dietary Wellness," your chances of contracting colon cancer can be reduced by 60% by eating cabbage weekly. Dr. Saxon-Graham states that those who never consume cabbage were three times more likely to develop colon cancer. A Japanese study shows that people who ate cabbage had the lowest fatality rate from any cancer. Therapeutic benefits have also been attributed to cabbage in relation to scurvy, gout, rheumatism (arthritis), eye diseases, asthma, pyorrhea and gangrene. See Raw Organic Vegetable Health Salad recipe page 73. We love cabbage and also we make a variety of sandwiches wrapped in cabbage leaves instead of bread.

For Arrhythmia and Heart Strengthening

The heart, a large muscular organ and your master pump uses large amounts of potassium to keep going strong for your entire life! It's the hardest working organ in the body (see below). It must have a constant, continuous supply of power and energy to continue beating. Apple cider vinegar contains a natural chemical that combines with heart fuel to make the heart muscle stronger and helps normalize blood pressure and cholesterol. Recent studies show apple cider vinegar helps remove dangerous artery plaque! To help blood pressure (see page 15) take Magnesium Orotate, the heart combo of CoQ10, Folic Acid, B6 and B12. Also enjoy your basic three apple cider vinegar drinks daily (see page 72 for recipe).

Let food be your medicine and medicine be your food. Nature heals: the physician is only nature's assistant. – Hippocrates, 400 B.C.

Every day the average heart, your best friend, beats 100,000 times and pumps 2,000 gallons of blood for nourishing your body. In about 70 years that adds up to more than 360 million (faithful) heartbeats. Please be good to your heart and live The Bragg Healthy Lifestyle for a long, happy, healthy life! Here's to Genesis 6:3 for you. – Patricia Bragg

Apple Cider Vinegar is Good for the Heart

As we age, we have become more susceptible to life-threatening diseases. According to the American Heart Association, about one out of every three adults has high blood pressure. Untreated this can bring on a deadly stroke or heart attack. Apple cider vinegar can aid in prevention of high blood pressure. The American Medical Association found potassium helps lowers blood pressure and hypertension.

Apple cider vinegar (made from fresh, organic apples) contains pectin, a soluble fiber, which aids in lowering cholesterol. Soluble fiber helps reduce cholesterol by binding with fiber, which your body then eliminates. This helps reduce heart risks, as in heart attacks and strokes.

ACV Helps Normalize Blood Pressure

Natural food acids served along with animal proteins are designed to lessen the blood thickening influence of these heavy proteins. In order for blood to circulate freely throughout the body, it must be thin. When blood thickens, it strains the heart! The blood pressure then goes up and a host of other health problems begin. Remember, blood has to circulate all over the body through the arteries, blood vessels and tiny capillaries. It's impossible for blood to circulate freely through these hair-size pipes when it is thickened with too many heavy protein meals, fats, hardened oils, etc.

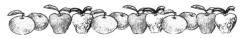

I started taking ACV and within days I noticed my blood pressure unbelievably lowered. I told all my friends in my community and bought a bottle of ACV for close friends. – Dr. Qasim Hussain Shah, Malaysia

---

Man is fully responsible for his nature and lifestyle. – Jean-Paul Sartre

---

Evidence reveals raw, organic apple cider vinegar has been shown to lower blood pressure and strengthen the heart muscles because it acts as a blood thinner, plaque remover and reduces the risk of strokes and heart attacks. It also contains important potassium and enzymes which are vital and needed to keep the heart and bloodstream healthy.

Several years ago, we met a woman with very high blood pressure. We put her on a two day apple cider vinegar, honey and water fast program with nothing to eat for 48 hours. She had an ACV drink five times daily, plus five glasses of pure distilled water = total of 10 glasses. In 48 hours, her blood pressure dropped to almost normal! The buzzing in her ears ceased, and her dull headache stopped. After a short period of correct eating (no salt, sugar, saturated fats, tea, coffee, etc.) combined with The Bragg Healthy Lifestyle, Fasting and the Apple Cider Vinegar Program, her blood pressure was normal and she felt reborn!

Fighting Diabetes with ACV

Taking apple cider vinegar before a meal is beneficial to people with diabetes. Over 86 million Americans are pre-diabetic and 30 million Americans have diabetes. Studies (see next page) have shown taking 1-2 tsps. ACV before meals is proven to dramatically reduce insulin and glucose spikes in the blood. These spikes can also cause Heart Disease in people with Type 2 Diabetes!

16

Research Reveals ACV Beneficial for Diabetes

The number of Americans with Type 2 Diabetes is expected to increase by 50% in the next 25 years. Organic apple cider vinegar can benefit people who are prediabetic or diabetic. Many doctors don't know about its beneficial effects. A study conducted at Arizona State University Department of Nutrition headed by Carol Johnston, Ph.D., R.D. and her colleagues showed that when apple cider vinegar is taken with a meal, it is effective in helping improve blood glucose and insulin levels by reducing the Glycemic Index of Foods. This research was published in *Diabetes Care,* the official journal of the American Diabetes Association. This research confirms the health benefits that apple cider vinegar can have for diabetics and for weight loss.

YOUR DAILY HABITS FORM YOUR FUTURE: Habits can be right or wrong, good or bad, healthy or unhealthy, rewarding or unrewarding. The right or wrong habits, decisions, actions, words or deeds . . . are up to you! Wisely choose your habits, as they can make or break your life! – Patricia Bragg

The authors of the study concluded, *"These data indicate that vinegar can significantly improve postprandial insulin sensitivity in insulin-resistant subjects . . . thus, vinegar may create physiological effects similar to acarbose or metformin (the two leading diabetic medications)."*

Study Shows Apple Cider Vinegar Benefits for Adults at Risk of Type 2 Diabetes

This pioneering research done by Dr. Carol Johnston, was inspired by Bragg Live Food Products to develop a line of vinegar drinks that would make it convenient to have organic apple cider vinegar available in a dose similar to what produced successful results in the study.

Johnston conducted another study at Arizona State University researching the benefits of apple cider vinegar that helps prevent Type 2 Diabetes. This time, participants drank Bragg Organic Apple Cider Vinegar Drinks, as a source of vinegar, sweetened with organic herb stevia extract. With 2 ACV servings in each 16-ounce bottle, test subjects drank the equivalent of one Tbsp of organic ACV twice daily with their meal. They drank the Bragg Organic ACV Drinks daily for a period of 12 weeks.

The results indicated that ingesting a Tbsp of organic ACV diluted in water twice a day at mealtime can help to lower the glycemic index of that meal.✱ This is due to the fact that acetic acid, an organic acid found naturally in apple cider vinegar, may be effective in inhibiting the enzyme that converts starch into simple sugars! This has beneficial effects on blood glucose concentrations in adults at risk for Type 2 Diabetes. It helps keep the blood glucose under control and helps to improve the insulin response to carbohydrates in meals. It is also beneficial to people who are trying to lose weight because a diet that is lower on the glycemic index will help with weight control as well! The authors of this study stated, "These data indicate that vinegar, a simple addition to meals, has anti-glycemic effects in adults at risk for Type 2 Diabetes."

✱ *Dr. Johnston, C.S. et al., Vinegar ingestion at mealtime reduced fasting glucose concentrations in healthy adults at risk for Type 2 Diabetes. – "Journal of Functional Foods" (2013)*

ACV Miracle for Overweight

50% of American adults are trying to lose weight. Over $65 billion dollars are spent yearly on diet programs and products. Rather than a yo-yo diet, these people need The Bragg Healthy Lifestyle and apple cider vinegar (ACV)! Please understand ACV will not reduce a person's weight who doesn't control their food intake! But the ACV drink and a healthy diet of 1,200 calories daily, plus regular exercise will do miracles in reducing excess weight.* Take this fat flushing ACV drink 3 times daily, see page 72. Also the Diet Research Center in England reported this:*"better reducing and firming with ACV daily massage (mix: 3 parts apple cider vinegar to 1 part organic olive oil in a bottle) helps the body reduce fat and cellulite."*

Along with this healthy ACV drink, there must be a healthy reducing diet. The best diet should consist of a wide variety of fresh organic fruits, veggies; raw salads and sprouts; raw nuts and seeds; raw, steamed, baked and stir-fried veggies; brown rice; whole grain pastas; tofu and beans. This means that all refined, processed, sugared products and beverages and dairy products are eliminated from your diet (see "Foods to Avoid" page 66).

Organic Apple Cider Vinegar: A Safer Way to Lose Weight

Chemical appetite suppressants and diet aids are flooding the market! Many have caused serious health problems and even death! Millions are searching for more natural ways to lose unwanted pounds and raw organic apple cider vinegar is getting results! Pectin found in apples is one of the benefits attributed to the correlation between apple cider vinegar and weight loss. Pectin, a natural fiber, helps clean out your digestive tract, plus the acidic nature of ACV helps stimulate bodily response that burns stored fat that accelerates weight loss!

My Fat Flush Plan uses raw organic apple cider vinegar as a prime ingredient for seasoning and even for cooking foods. We find that blood sugar levels become normalized and individuals can digest protein so much more effectively with apple cider vinegar.
– Ann Louise Gittleman, Ph.D., C.N.S., author, "Fat Flush Plan"

Fighting Fat with ACV

Thermogenic herbs suppress appetite: barley green, spirulina, kelp, sea vegetables, green drinks, etc. Also take on an empty stomach before bed and early rising 500 mg L-Carnitine and 200-400 mcg Chromium Picolinate to promote weight loss and firming. Along with portion controlled meals, fasting, exercise and ACV drinks, these herbs can help.

Combatting Underweight

Raw apple cider vinegar is proving to be one of the greatest health aids known to science. It's a 100% natural substance produced by powerful natural enzymes from healthy organic apples, free of any toxic chemicals!

The underweight person is usually deficient in these powerful enzymes and therefore cannot use or burn up the food that is put into their body. No matter how much fatty food, protein or any other kind of food is ingested, often it is not used properly by the body if important enzymes are missing. Enzyme deficiencies always cause problems! If underweight, drink the following ACV drink each morning upon arising: 2 tsps. ACV and 2 tsps. honey in a glass of distilled water. Add to this 2 drops of liquid iodine made from seaweed, available in Health Stores. Adding natural iodine is important to the thyroid and body health and helps normalize body weight up or down as needed. Then, with each meal take a multi-digestive enzyme and always be faithful to The Bragg Healthy Lifestyle. Remember, healthy foods are needed body fuel to enjoy a healthy, long, fulfilled life.

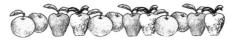

Millions of people every year pay thousands of dollars for state-of-the-art testing to learn their risk for heart disease. However, experts say fresh vegetables and a health club membership may be better buys than lab tests. People who eat a diet low in fat and cholesterol and rich in plant foods, who don't smoke, who exercise regularly, keep weight and blood pressure in normal ranges are less likely to have a heart attack than those who don't take precautions. – Harvard Health Letter • Health.Harvard.edu

How to Improve the Digestion

Millions suffer indigestion (gerd), which is aggravated by poor digestion and weak saliva juices. This causes distress – gas, heartburn, burping and stomach bloating. Before mealtime, sip $^1/3$ tsp. apple cider vinegar with equal parts water. Hold in mouth for a minute before swallowing. This promotes enzymes and saliva, which improves digestion that starts in the mouth. This causes stomach digestive fluids to flow faster, resulting in improved digestion and better health. ACV also protects against food borne pathogens.

Apple Cider Vinegar and Constipation

It's important the bowels move easily and regularly! Outgo should equal intake. You should have a bowel movement soon after arising and within an hour after meals. Flaxseeds and its' tea with ACV act as bowel lubricants, as do prunes, fresh fruits, vegetables and distilled water.

20

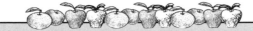

Make this ACV-Flaxseed Bowel Lubricant Cleanse Tea

Boil 2 cups distilled water with 4 Tbsps whole flaxseeds for 15 minutes or soak overnight. (Mixture becomes jelly-like when cold.) Stir 2 Tbsps of this mixture, plus 1 tsp. ACV in 8 oz. distilled (hot or cold) water. Add maple syrup or honey if desired. Drink upon arising and an hour before bed. Store mixture in refrigerator and use when needed.

Flaxseeds are packed with omega-3, lignans and fiber, which are natural antioxidants. Omega-3 helps remove toxins and prevent heart disease. Lignans provide up to 700 times the amount of fiber found in legumes or whole grains. Whole flaxseeds can be stored for months in an airtight container in a cool, dark place. Grind them in a coffee grinder as needed.

Organic apple cider vinegar with the "mother" is vital to the body's digestive balance by stimulating flow of precious enzymes and saliva in the mouth. I recommend it to stop heartburn, indigestion, gerd, gas and to improve digestion: sip $^1/3$ tsp. ACV with water before meals to activate the flow of digestive juices. – Gabriel Cousens, M.D., author, "Conscious Eating"

For Healthy Elimination: Use miracle psyllium husk powder. Add 1 Tbsp of this cleansing herb to any of these: Apple Cider Vinegar Drink (see page 72), juice, distilled water, herb tea, soups, etc.; let it soak for 2 minutes before drinking or eating! This helps cleanse mucus along small intestine and colon walls and pulls toxins from intestinal tract. Also use organic, extra-virgin olive oil over salads, veggies, potatoes, etc. – it helps elimination and detoxifies the colon, plus adds delicious flavor to foods.

To Check Bowel Elimination Time: Have some organic fresh or frozen whole corn with your evening meal. But purposely don't chew all the kernels. (Always chew food thoroughly otherwise.) Check stools to see when corn is eliminated, usually within 14 hours. When it's cleansed of toxins and malnutrition is treated, the body becomes healthier and more normal! Because constipation brings on serious health problems, including arthritis, it's important to keep the pipes (colon and arteries) clean and open by faithfully following The Bragg Healthy Lifestyle.

21

For Easier-Flowing Bowel Movements:

It's natural to squat to have bowel movements. It opens up the anal area more directly. When on toilet, putting feet up 6-8" on waste basket or footstool provides the same squatting effect. Now raise arms, stretch hands above head so the transverse colon can push to empty with ease. It's important for you to drink 8 to 10 glasses pure water daily – works miracles! After dinner take 1 psyllium husk veg. capsule daily or do Flaxseed Cleanse, on page 20.

The body is 75% water (see chart on page 95) and pure, steam-distilled (chemical-free) water is important for total health. Drink 8-10 glasses of water and ACV drinks daily. Read *Water – The Shocking Truth*, and read pages 93-98 for more information on the importance of distilled water. See pages 137-140 for Patricia Bragg Health Books.

Fasting gives rest to digestion, assimilation and body's vital organs.

Fight Kidney and Bladder Problems

Avoid all animal, dairy, salt, coffee, alcohol and sugar products. All ages should follow The Bragg Healthy Lifestyle for optimum health. Use ACV on salads and have your ACV drink 3 times daily. ACV can help bladder problems and dissolve some types of stones. Drink 8 glasses of distilled water, plus some organic, unsweetened cranberry juice. Add $1/3$ tsp. ACV to each glass, which helps acidify urine, inhibits bacterial growth and promotes healing. You may sweeten cranberry drink with organic grape juice, raw honey or herb Stevia. You can also do 2-3 day watermelon only flush. Thoroughly chew or grind the seeds, too. This is a great kidney and bladder cleanser and healer!

For bed-wetting: Mix and sip $1/2$ to 1 tsp. buckwheat honey with $1/2$ tsp. ACV before bedtime. It's best to stop liquids 3 hours before bedtime, except for small sips.

For all kidney and bladder problems: Children and adults should drink 6-8 glasses of distilled water daily. It's important for urinary tract and kidneys. Have ACV drink (page 72) and this healing hot drink: 2 Tbsps. dried corn silk to 1 quart distilled water or try marshmallow herb tea, 2 to 3 times daily. Add $1/2$ tsp. ACV to each cup and sweeten with 1 tsp. buckwheat honey. (Save dry corn silks from fresh corn and store in airtight bottle.)

To soothe and heal bladder infections: Add 1 cup ACV to warm low sitz-bath. Use 1 to 2 times daily. Use a Dipstick self-tester from drugstore to check if you have a urinary tract infection.*

To eliminate "dribbles": To keep bladder sphincter muscles tightened and toned – urinate – stop – urinate – stop, 4 times, twice daily when voiding. This simple Kegel exercise works. After age of 40, do every day. (*www.prevention.com/health/how-do-kegel-exercises*)

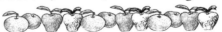

IMPORTANT: We don't endorse antibiotics, but if you ever take them, please take 'Lactobacillus Acidophilus' liquid or capsules. Acidophilus helps replace the friendly bacteria in your body.

Learning is a treasure that will follow its owner everywhere. – Chinese Proverb

Apple Cider Vinegar Combats Gallstones

Before starting this two day gallbladder flush, prepare for one week by drinking slowly – upon arising, mid-morning, mid-afternoon and after dinner – $1/2$ tsp. ACV with a 6 oz. glass of apple juice; or if hypoglycemic or diabetic, then dilute with half distilled water. Organic, unfiltered apple juice is rich in malic acid, potassium, pectins and enzymes. These act as solvents to soften and help remove debris (small stones) and cleanse your body. Doctors have non-surgical methods for removing difficult, larger stones using sound waves! But it's best to purge small and medium-sized ones twice yearly as they can grow to cause problems! (See testimonies below and on top of page D.)

During two-day gallbladder flush no food is eaten, only liquids. Combine in 8 oz glass: $1/3$ cup organic extra-virgin olive oil (no substitutes), $2/3$ cup organic apple juice and 1 tsp. organic ACV with the 'mother.' Drink mixture three times the first day. *At night, sleep on your right side when on flush, pulling right knee toward chest to open pathway.* On second day, take mixture twice. On both days drink all the organic apple juice desired, but no water or any other liquid. (*This gallbladder flush is not for diabetics unless supervised by a health professional.*)

About midmorning on the third day, eat a raw variety salad (nature's broom) of cabbage, carrots, celery, beets, tomatoes, sprouts and lettuce, with lots of ACV and olive oil. If desired, have a bowl of lightly steamed greens: kale, collards, chard or any leafy greens. Season with ACV and squeeze of lemon – this gives delicious flavor to greens.

This Gallbladder Flush saved me from having gallbladder surgery. Praise God I discovered the amazing health miracles organic apple cider vinegar brings. I travel around the world and love being a Health Crusader. – Kari Isaeff, Santa Barbara, CA

Your book "Apple Cider Vinegar" saved me from having my gallbladder out. The specialist wanted to take my gallbladder out, instead I followed your apple cider vinegar flush and it worked along with healing prayers at church! I think all book and health stores should carry your vinegar book. I am grateful for you writing it. God Bless You. – Carmen Puro, Michigan

We take this miracle cleanser flush at least once or twice a year. Check your bowel movements for tiny, greenish-brown stones. This flush will amaze you what your gallbladder, stomach and colon will clean out!

When on flush nausea may occur. This shows toxins, mucus and bile are being dumped in the stomach. Your body wants it out! If nauseated, your body is saying: "Drink 1 to 2 glasses of purified water and regurgitate until your stomach is empty." (You might have to depress your tongue while leaning over the bowl.) Once it's out, you will feel better right away! Remember, it's always the wisest decision when nauseated to get out whatever is causing an upset stomach.

Apple Cider Vinegar Helps Shrink Prostate

With a fork, "whip" 2 Tbsps. apple cider vinegar with 2 Tbsps. organic olive oil and a dash of cinnamon. Use this ACV mixture daily over salads, sliced tomatoes, avocados and steamed veggies. Enjoy with meals, zinc-rich raw pumpkin seeds. Also take Zinc, Prostex and Saw Palmetto supplements which are healers for the prostate.

Apple Cider Vinegar for Female Troubles

- **Bath:** Add 2 cups ACV to water. **Sitz-Bath:** Add 1 cup.
- **To help with Hot Flashes, PMS, UTI:** drink Apple Cider Vinegar Drink 3-5 times daily, see pages 72.
- **To shrink, tighten or tone flabby stomach muscles:** Daily do Kegel and Bragg Posture Exercise (page 88). Fast one day weekly, (page 105) and do exercise faithfully. Eat daily Raw Organic Vegetable Salad (page 73).

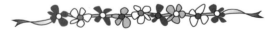

TEMPORARY RELIEF OF PAIN ASSOCIATED WITH MENSTRUAL CRAMPS: At onset of pain apply a compress prepared as follows: Soak washcloth in solution of 1 cup ACV and 1 cup warm water. Ring out cloth, place on abdomen, then put hot water bottle on top of compress and cover with towel 15-30 minutes. Repeat as needed. – Dr. Shalini Kapoor, N.D., MPH

Avoid all self-drugging, such as aspirin and similar drugs, pain-killers, sleeping pills, tranquilizers, antihistamines, laxatives, strong cathartics, fizzing bromides, etc. You are not qualified to prescribe drugs for yourself. The side-effects and results can be serious! – Patricia Bragg

Apple Cider Vinegar and Arthritis

People ask if ACV cures arthritis. This is not possible, for curing is an internal biological function that only the body can perform! We have seen miracles how the ACV drink helps fight arthritis. A healthy diet with ACV, exercise, deep breathing, rest and living The Bragg Healthy Lifestyle are required to put the body in a condition to cure itself! ACV is an important part of this program (page 45). When all Mother Nature's supreme forces are used, the body will turn from sickness to wellness. Super health is something you must desire, seek out, earn and always guard and treasure for your life's sake!

Fight Arthritis with Apple Cider Vinegar

Hard, stony deposits fill up, cement, enlarge and cripple joints! Crippling, painful arthritis and joint problems are the sad result! Flush out stony crystals with your daily ACV drinks. Upon arising, an hour before lunch, and before dinner have delicious ACV drink (page 72) as follows:

Add 1-2 tsps. equally of apple cider vinegar and raw honey (diabetics use Stevia) in 8 oz glass of distilled water. Also add ACV to salads and steamed greens. Be faithful to The Bragg Healthy Lifestyle and 24-hour fasts. Eat 60% to 70% healthy, raw foods (organic is best), drink 8 glasses daily of distilled water. To help heal and regenerate, take a natural multi-vitamin and minerals, Glucosamine, Chondroitin and MSM supplements, and 1-2 tsps. cod liver oil daily!

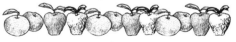

You are a Miracle – Self-Cleansing, Self-Repairing, Self-Healing –
Please become aware of "YOU" and be thankful for all your
miracle blessings that take place daily! – Paul C. Bragg, N.D., Ph.D.

A heart is not judged by how much you love, but by how much
you are loved by others. – The Wizard of Oz to the Tin Man

The future belongs to those who believe in the beauty of their dreams.
– Eleanor Roosevelt, wife of President Franklin D. Roosevelt, 1933 – 1945

Toxic Acid Arthritic Crystals Make Joints Grind

The grinding sound you hear in your neck when you roll your head is the toxic arthritic acid crystals that have deposited themselves on the uppermost bone of your spine – the Atlas. Just as ACV washes sludge off windows, it also washes the body sludge from the joints and cardiovascular system of the body. Fasting, and taking the Apple Cider Vinegar Drink (page 72) will help eliminate acid crystals from the joints. A feeling of agelessness gradually will replace that tight, stiff, ageing feeling. You will start to feel more flexible, pain-free and loose in every moveable joint of your body.

All Through Life You Fight Acid Crystals

When acid crystals harden in the joints and tissues, the joints become stiff, and tissues age and harden. Also meat becomes tough and tasteless. When animals are given apple cider vinegar regularly, the precipitated acid crystals enter into a solution and then pass out of the body, thus making the body tissues healthier and tender. This applies to human flesh also. Now, when body tissues hold all the precipitated acid crystals they can, the crystals then appear in the bursae and the joints of the body, resulting in bursitis and arthritis. 1 to 2 tsps. apple cider vinegar with 1 to 2 tsps. raw honey in a glass of distilled water three times daily (page 72), helps relieve stiff, aching, prematurely old joints. You be the judge. See how elastic and flexible all your joints become!

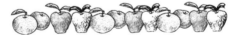

I started using organic apple cider vinegar and have never felt better. My joint pain and stiffness is fast disappearing and my energy level has improved. I am sold on it for life. Thank You! – Joseph M. Cole

For pain and stiffness, arthritis, osteoarthritis and to help heal and regenerate cartilage and bones, use boron supplements, glucosamine, and chondroitin sulfates and MSM combo works miracles!

I will praise Thee, for I am fearfully and wonderfully made. Marvellous are Thy works and that my soul shall knoweth right. – Psalms 139:14

Caution: The Army Diet – what you overeat goes to the front.

Keep Your Joints and Tissues Youthful

Sadly, most people have lost normal contact with Mother Nature and simple, natural living! They no longer know how to eat the simple way intended. If you suffer from prematurely old joints and hardened tissues, be sure to take the ACV mixture three times daily. Eliminate or cut down on animal proteins. Stop all refined sugars, products and beverages! Soon you will see how youthful your body and joints begin to feel!

Take This 48 Hour Test

For 2 full days, take nothing into your system but liquids. Have the ACV drink 3 to 5 times daily, plus another 4 to 5 glasses of distilled water daily as well. Ample water is needed to flush the toxins out!

On the second and third day, after you have eaten nothing else for 48 hours, take a sample of your first morning urine and store in labeled bottles with tight lids. Keep on shelf for 2 weeks, then examine sediment at bottom of bottles. These are some of the disease-causing toxins that were thankfully flushed out of your body!

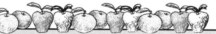

Healthy Mind Habits Promote Health and Longevity

Wake up and say – "Today I am going to be happier, healthier and wiser in my daily living! I am the captain of my life and am going to steer it living a 100% healthy lifestyle!" FACT: Happy people look younger, are healthier and live longer! – Patricia Bragg

Don't regret ageing gracefully and living longer.
It's a privilege denied to many.

If I had to give up everything health related and keep only one item – organic apple cider vinegar would be the one! At 35 years old, I felt like 95. I could hardly get through a day without going to bed in the afternoon. I tried everything and nothing helped. My wife's Grandpa "took an ACV nip" every morning and lived a long and active life, despite having smoked for a large part of his life. I also remember my Great Nana doing it. I tried it and in no time started feeling healthier and stronger! I am almost 37 now and have not been sick in over a year. I tell everyone about organic apple cider vinegar and have given over 20 bottles away to my family and friends. Thank You!! – Dave Streen, Williams Bay, WI

Potassium – The Master Mineral

Always keep in mind the fact that potassium puts toxic poisons in solution so they can be flushed out of the body. **The body is self-cleansing, self-correcting, self-repairing and self-healing!** Just give it the tools to work with and soon it will help you enjoy a painless, tireless, ageless body, regardless of age! Forget age and calendar years, for age isn't toxic! You age prematurely when you suffer from malnutrition and potassium deficiencies. These cause low Vital Force, toxic waste buildups and poor elimination that allow disease to proliferate!

The Bragg Healthy Lifestyle will help you rebuild your Vital Force. Watch the transformation that will take place in your body when you faithfully follow your ACV regimen. You can and will create the kind of person you want to be! Plan, plot and follow through! Start now!

Although you must follow this program closely, please don't try to do everything listed immediately. Remember, it took you a long time of living by wrong habits to cause any of the problems your body might have now. So, it's going to take time for the body to cleanse, repair and rebuild itself into a more *perfect healthy home* for you! Please remember, your body is your temple while on this earth, so cherish it and protect it!

What Becomes of the Acid Crystals Precipitated in the Body That Age Us?

When you think of "old" people you usually think of them as having stiffness in their body, with tough, brittle flesh (see Dr. Carrel's study on page 9). Why do people get stiff in the joints and their flesh tough when they have added birthdays to their life? Most people would answer this complex question with the remark, "Because they are old." But this isn't the real answer why people get stiff joints and tough flesh.

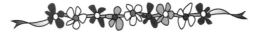

Anyone who stops learning is old – whether 20 or 80. Anyone who keeps learning stays more youthful. The greatest thing in life is to keep your mind and heart young! – Henry Ford • www.TheHenryFord.org

The answer to premature ageing is unhealthy living and potassium deficiency! People rarely study their bodies or learn what to eat for healthy tissues and youthful joints (ACV brings miracles). They're satisfied to eat what they think agrees with them. Or they eat foods they were reared on as children and carry these early eating habits (sadly often unhealthy) right into their adult life and then into their children's lives!

ACV Helps Banish Stiffness From Body

You will find, after several months of the ACV and honey drink taken 3 times daily – that the stiffness and misery will be gone from your joints and body. You will discover you can walk or run up stairs without any effort and pain. Follow Natural Healthy Laws on page 47. You will notice that you look, act and feel younger!

Make The Bragg Healthy Lifestyle a life-long daily habit! Over the years we have seen many stiff-jointed, prematurely old people transform themselves into new, youthful, healthy people! We can't do it for you! You must make the effort to give apple cider vinegar and The Bragg Healthy Lifestyle a chance to prove what they can do for you!

WISE HEALTH ADVISE FROM DR. DEAN ORNISH: We tend to think of advances in medicine as being a new drug, new surgical technique, new laser, something high-tech and expensive. We often have a hard time believing the simple choices we make each day in our diet and lifestyle can make such a powerful difference in the quality and quantity of our lives, but they most often do. My health program consists of four main parts: exercise, nutrition, stress management, love and support. These promote not only living longer, but living better. – ornish.com.

The body must obey your strong, wise mind. Flesh is dumb! You can put anything in your stomach from coffee to hot dogs. It is not the stomach that rules the body, but your intelligent and reasoning mind! A properly-directed mind can inspire the body to faithfully follow The Bragg Healthy Lifestyle, thereby helping the body to become closer to physical healthy perfection.

If you can't do great things, do small things in a great way.
– Napoleon Hill

ACV Helps Relieve Muscle Cramps

Many people are awakened in the middle of the night with sharp, painful muscle cramps. These often occur in the feet and lower or upper legs. Sometimes they occur in the stomach, intestines and occasionally in the heart. These are frightening experiences! Most people who experience leg cramps are forced to jump out of bed, stomp and firmly massage area to get relief. When precipitated acid crystals get into the circulation of legs and other body parts, they can cause severe cramps. We recommend taking 2 tsps. ACV and 1-2 tsps. honey (page 72) in glass distilled water three times daily to relieve these painful cramps. This allows precipitated toxic acid crystals to enter into a solution and pass out of the body, causing cramps to cease. Calcium and also magnesium orotate taken one hour before bedtime also help prevent cramping, plus help promote a sounder sleep. Also ACV baths help, see below.

ACV Bath and Massage Can Soothe Muscle Soreness, Cramps and Aching Joints

To soothe aching muscles, cramps and joints, there's nothing like an ACV bath combined with a bath self-massage! While soaking in a warm bath with 1 cup ACV added, massage entire body, starting at feet. Gently squeeze and relax each part of the foot, working slowly up right leg to hip, then left leg. Continue up torso, arms and neck, always rubbing toward the heart. For the face, lightly stroke skin in upward direction; avoid pulling facial skin down. Finish with firm fingertip dry massage in circular motions over the scalp, then finger rub your entire ears.

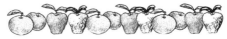

Raw, organic apple cider vinegar with the mother enzyme is healthy because it's loaded with vitamins, minerals and is rich in potassium. Apple cider vinegar helps balance the body's vital acid/alkaline balance.
"Do As I Do . . . Drink organic apple cider vinegar drink 3 times daily!"
– Julian Whitaker, M.D., Health & Healing Newsletter • DrWhitaker.com

The first wealth is your health. – Ralph Waldo Emerson

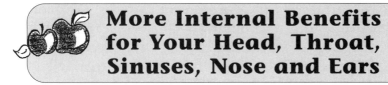
Apple Cider Vinegar Relieves Headaches

People blame their headaches on many different organs of the body. Most headaches are blamed on the eyes, the nerves, the liver, the sinuses, the stomach, the bowel, kidneys or allergies and even the climate. Headaches can be put into two different classifications:

One type of chronic headache can be associated with toxic buildup and illness! A headache is an alarm telling the person that deep down in their body, destruction is going on. Pain and headaches are Mother Nature's great red flashing warning signal to take fast action! There may be trouble anywhere throughout the body. It could be in the liver, gallbladder, kidneys, bowel or any of the body's organs. It may be related to or caused by sensitive sinus, allergy, or alcohol problems, etc. See pages 105-110 to detox.

31

The second type of headache is emotional! This is often caused by nervousness, anxiety, stress, strain, tension or any personal or emotional upsets! This is a world where we must be associated with other human beings. Your daily life with others can throw you into many upsetting emotional problems because they can arouse emotions of fear, jealousy, envy, hate, greed, self-pity or self-indulgence! When emotions reach a boiling point, you can usually end up with a dull, throbbing headache. The worst headache is the migraine, which causes the sufferer to feel as if their head is splitting. **Read these Patricia Bragg Books for more Health Guides:** *The Miracle of Fasting; Bragg Back & Foot Fitness Program; Building Powerful Nerve Force & Positive Energy;* and *The Bragg Healthy Lifestyle.* See booklist pages 137-140.

Avoid These Foods That Can Trigger Headaches and Migraines

- Additive and chemical-laced foods
- Caffeine-containing foods
- Salty, sugary or wheat-based foods
- Condiments, sulfites, MSG
- Dairy foods, especially cheese
- Alcohol and diet sodas

– Linda Page, N.D., Ph.D., author of "Healthy Healing"

We have found in our many years of research on all kinds of headaches that when the body triggers a headache, the urine is alkaline rather than the normal acid. The kidneys are disturbed by the emotions and it means the body is off-balance! The fast working malic acid of apple cider vinegar can help relieve headaches by aiding the kidneys to return urine to normal (average 6.4 pH) acidity.

Vaporized ACV can also help relieve headaches. In a vaporizer or small pan, put 2 Tbsps. of ACV, 1 drop of Oil of Oregano in 2 cups of purified water. Bring this mixture to a boil. As the vapor begins to rise, turn heat off, put a towel over your head, lean over the steam, taking five deep slow breaths of the steam vapors. Also try hot and cold vinegar compresses to your forehead and neck area, then do some shoulder/neck rolls and firmly massage neck, head and shoulders, and if needed visit your Chiropractor. For pain use Bromelain 500 mg (available at health stores) – it acts like aspirin without the toxic stomach upset. Many chronic headache sufferers have told us they get blessed relief with this method. By doing these things and faithfully following The Bragg Healthy Lifestyle, soon you will have no need for commercial headache remedies and pain killers!

Apple Cider Vinegar Zaps Sore Throat and Laryngitis

Organic, raw ACV is a dangerous enemy to all kinds of germs that attack the throat and mouth! To fight the germs and keep the throat healthy, an ACV gargle mixture works miracles (1 tsp. to $1/2$ glass water). Gargle three mouthfuls of mixture each hour, then spit it out. Don't swallow the gargled mixture, because ACV acts like a sponge, drawing out throat and mouth germs and toxins. As the throat feels better, gargle every three hours. We have rock and roll bands to Metropolitan Opera famous singers, the youthful Beach Boys, Bette Midler and Carrie Underwood using apple cider vinegar to keep their throats healthy and germ-free. It's important for singers, teachers, ministers, public speakers and you!

I love and use ACV daily. This is my secret of all secrets. – Katy Perry, singer

Along with gargling, we use an ACV wet compress as follows: first, place a thin ACV-soaked cloth over your throat area, cover with Saran Wrap, then use a flat hot water bag or moist, hot wrung-out towel to heat the area, allowing ACV to absorb through the skin. This ACV hot compress is also great for cleansing and healing your chest area when treating all lung congestions: colds, flu, bronchitis, emphysema, chest pains and asthma! It feels good, too!

Even in good health, use ACV gargle twice weekly to remove any body toxins being eliminated through the throat tissues. The gargle is also helpful during fasting, when the throat may produce a stringy mucus as part of detoxifying process: Read *The Miracle of Fasting* book, it contains the powerful health message of fasting to detox, cleanse and renew the body. See pages 105-110 and 138.

Apple Cider Vinegar Combats Mucus

Millions have postnasal drip and are plagued with mucus in their lungs, sinus cavities, nose and throat. If mucus sufferers remove all dairy products and sugars from diet, follow The Bragg Healthy Lifestyle, take a weekly 24-hour fast and use ample ACV, soon mucus conditions will vanish on this healthy toxicless and mucusless diet!

Oil of Oregano – Nature's Versatile Healer and Detox

Oil of Oregano is a very powerful herbal body defender and cleanser and it is used to fight: viruses; flus; colds; allergies; asthma; E. coli; Salmonella; parasitic yeast and bacterial infections; upset stomach; menstrual problems; urinary tract problems and arthritis. Take with food. Available in capsules or drops at your health and vitamin stores. (When needed for winter cold maintenance do the *Breathing Detox* below.)

Breathing Detox: Place 2-3 drops of "Oil of Oregano" in 2 quarts of boiling water. Put a towel over your head, breathe in the vapors through your mouth and then your nose. It's powerful, so close your eyes! This opens up your lungs to remove congestion. Relieves colds, flu, and bronchitis congestion. Do as needed 1-3 times daily.

ACV Mouthwash: add 1 tsp. of ACV to an 8 oz. glass of purified water – kills mouth bacteria, fights plaque and tartar. Promotes healing and helps prevent gum disease.

Post Nasal Drip: Upon arising, have a glass of warm distilled water with 1-2 tsps. of ACV and 1-2 tsps. raw honey (recipe page 72). Enjoy this mid-morning and mid-afternoon.

Throat/Mucus gargle: Add 1 tsp. of ACV to a glass of warm water to help clean out mucus. Do 3 times daily until mucus subsides. Along with ACV drinks, enjoy fresh carrot and green juices between meals. It's important to sip fresh juices slowly, as they are really foods, not beverages. Small amounts of juice (or food) in your mouth at one time will be better digested and more easily used by the body chemistry.

Apple Cider Vinegar for Nose Bleeds

Besides bleeding from an injury, nosebleeds can be caused by low humidity in your home or office, colds, allergies, low levels of vitamin K, chronic sinusitis, high altitudes, excessive heat and some medications.

ACV is useful in getting a nosebleed to stop. Soak small cotton ball or gauze in ACV and lightly pack in nostrils. Relax, sit down and lean forward 10 minutes (breathe through mouth) pressing nostrils together while ACV pack helps blood congeal. Repeat if needed. You can also pour some vinegar on a cloth and wash neck, nose and temples with it. Vitamins C, K and Rutin are helpful. Be sure to drink 8-10 glasses of pure water daily – nosebleeds are often caused by dehydration. (web: *Health911.com/nosebleeds*)

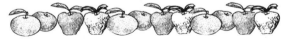

"Breathe Deep Yogi Tea" *helps clear breathing passages and nourish lung tissues. This healing formula utilizes licorice, basil, cinnamon, ginger and peppermint to loosen phlegm and relax muscles of respiratory tract.*

A large percent of sinus problems are caused by bacteria and pollutants, such as smoke, dust and the overuse of nasal decongestant medication.

I give thanks each day for all the miracle blessings I receive daily.
– Patricia Bragg

ACV for Ear Infections and Ear Aches

Causes of ear infections are many and home treatments can soothe painful symptoms and hasten healing. Causes range from a foreign object or insect in your ear, to wax buildup or bacteria. If ear pain remains, a doctor should be consulted. **Never place liquids in an ear with a broken eardrum.**

ACV helps chronic inflammation, middle ear infections, ear aches, ear blockages and swimmer's ear, a condition from swimming and showering. ACV changes pH of the ear canal, creating an environment where bacteria and viruses cannot thrive. Dilute ACV with equal parts distilled water and put 3-4 drops into ear (lie on side to let soak in). Repeat several times a day. Make sure liquid is room temperature. Drug stores stock ear dropper syringes. If ear and skin problems persist, it is best to see a health professional (web: *LiveStrong.com*).

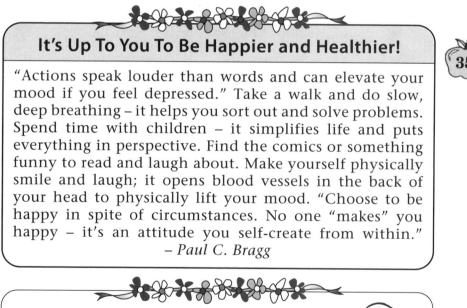

It's Up To You To Be Happier and Healthier!

35

"Actions speak louder than words and can elevate your mood if you feel depressed." Take a walk and do slow, deep breathing – it helps you sort out and solve problems. Spend time with children – it simplifies life and puts everything in perspective. Find the comics or something funny to read and laugh about. Make yourself physically smile and laugh; it opens blood vessels in the back of your head to physically lift your mood. "Choose to be happy in spite of circumstances. No one "makes" you happy – it's an attitude you self-create from within."
– *Paul C. Bragg*

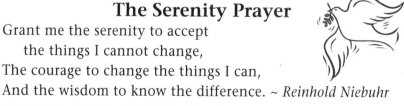

The Serenity Prayer

Grant me the serenity to accept
the things I cannot change,
The courage to change the things I can,
And the wisdom to know the difference. ~ *Reinhold Niebuhr*

"Read uplifting books and turn off the news. Just smiling can enhance your mood and health." – Kenneth R. Pelletier, Ph.D, M.D., Professor at UC San Francisco

Mother Nature Loves You To Enjoy Her Beauty

Let me look upward
into the branches
Of the towering oak
And know that it grew
slowly and well.

Give me, amidst
the confusion
of my day
The calmness of the
everlasting hills.

Let me pause
to look at a flower,
to smell a rose —
God's autograph,
to chat with a friend,
to read a few lines
from a good book.

Break the tensions
of my nerves
With the soothing music
of singing streams
and gentle rains
That live in
my memory.

Follow steps of the godly,
and stay on the right path
to enjoy life to the fullest.
— Proverbs 2:20-21

Open your eyes to behold wondrous things out of Thy law.
— Psalm 119:18

36

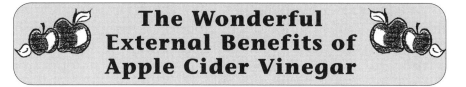
Apple Cider Vinegar for Healthy, Vibrant Skin

Reap vitality with the apple cider vinegar massage: To a small basin of warm distilled water, add $^1/_2$ cup of ACV. Dip both hands in mixture and massage this all over your body (in shower or bathtub): face, neck, chest, arms, shoulders, back, abdomen, legs and feet. Massage mixture on skin thoroughly, be gentle on face. This leaves skin soft and pH balanced. Healthy skin has an acid reaction, for it's throwing off toxic poisons through its billions of pores. **(Skin is often called your third kidney.)** After thoroughly wetting the skin with the mixture gently rub and massage until the skin is dry. Do this at least twice a week and do not wash it off; leave it on the body. As you massage the mixture into the skin, you will feel a new vitality coming into your body!

Also soaking in an ACV bath helps restore acid to alkaline balance in your body. If baths are not your thing, try mixing a cup of ACV and warm water in a spray bottle and spray yourself after a shower, rub it in and feel refreshed!

The reason this treatment is far better than using soap is because soap has an alkaline reaction on the skin and you don't want that! By keeping the skin in an acid reaction, it will help you have healthier skin. We've never used soap on our face or body, just ACV and it's worked wonders. If you use soap – use high quality organic soaps only.

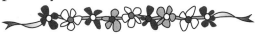

SAD FACTS: Many people go throughout life committing partial suicide – destroying their health, skin, heart, youth, beauty, talents, energies and creative qualities. Indeed, to learn how to be good to oneself is often more difficult than to learn how to be good to others. – Dr. Paul C. Bragg

---

It's supposed to be a professional secret, but I'll tell you anyway.
We doctors do nothing. We only help and encourage the doctor within.
– Albert Schweitzer, Nobel Peace Prize

We find after hard exercise or long mental work that we get a new feeling of strength and energy after one of these ACV massages. Also try gentle dry skin brushing with a loofah pad or vegetable brush next time you feel mentally or physically tired (page 117). It helps remove old skin cells and toxic wastes. We know you'll want to do it often. The health benefits of improved circulation are obvious!

ACV Cleanser and Toner for Skin Problems

To open your pores and loosen dirt and grease from your face, turn off heat under a pan of steaming ACV water (3 Tbsp. of ACV to a quart of purified water). Steam your face over pan and use a towel draped over your head to trap the steam. Afterwards pat ACV on face with a cotton ball to remove loosened dirt. Repeat steaming and cleansing twice. Then gently squeeze out any white/blackheads. Then pat or spray on chilled ACV toner (50% ACV and 50% distilled water mixture, keep in your refrigerator) to close pores and tone skin. Do steam cleansing weekly, as needed. Another excellent skin healer is aloe gel or try fresh aloe vera cactus pulp. Cut off 1 inch of aloe vera rib, slit open and rub yellowish pulp directly on skin. We grow our own aloe plants, you can grow them in pots also. Aloe is a great healer – gently dab on burns, pimples, cuts, bites, etc!

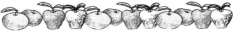

I have suffered from psoriasis and acne for 10 years. Since I started The Bragg Healthy Lifestyle and ACV program my skin looks better than ever. My rough spots are clearing and new skin is growing to replace the dry patches. Thank you, I am a Bragg Health Fan for Life!! – Cathrine Westergaard, NY

For over a year I was having terrible skin issues and doctors were no help. No medications or creams were helping. My skin was peeling like I had a sunburn all the time. After meeting you and using ACV as a tonic for my face, it cleared up to where you would never know I had a problem. Thank you for coming into my life when I needed help! Love & Blessings! – Becky, FL

I've been using raw, organic apple cider vinegar skin facial/spray and organic olive oil for 10 years instead of expensive skin care products. I'm 53 and my skin and face are soft and so youthful looking, people often ask me what I do. I tell them about vinegar and olive oil for their skin and body. Thank you so much! – Pat Williams, CA

Younger Looking Skin in Minutes With Apple Cider Vinegar Skin Tonic and Facial

The skin consists of microscopically small, flat scales that constantly flake off, revealing new skin beneath outer, older scale layers. Millions have old, tired, dead, dry outer scales that don't peel off promptly, slowing new growth and leaving skin dry, sallow, and lifeless.

• **ACV Facial:** first, wash your skin with warm water (no soap). Next, apply a wrung-out, hot water-soaked cloth to your face for three minutes, then remove. Now soak a thin cotton washcloth in hot ACV water (1 Tbsp. ACV per cup water) again apply to your face. Cover ACV-soaked washcloth with a cotton towel wrung out in hot water. Now lie down for 15 minutes or longer with your feet elevated up on a couch, against a wall, or use a slant board. This brings more blood circulation to revitalize your face for cell rejuvenation. Now remove both cloths and gently rub your skin upwards with coarse towel or our favorite – small loofah face pad. This rub removes the hundreds of old, dry skin scales that have been detached and loosened by the ACV facial.

You can repeat this ACV facial weekly or as needed. Your skin will look more youthful and will shine like a polished apple. We should all have pride in looking our best. You will be truly amazed and proud of yourself with the results from these age-reversing, simple to do health treatments!

• **ACV Skin Tonic Spray:** for men and women. Spray or pat in the am or pm on face (50% ACV and 50% distilled water mixture – keep in the refrigerator) daily for amazing results!

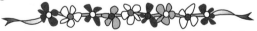

Don't procrastinate and keep waiting for "the right moment." Today – take action, plan, plot and follow through with your goals, dreams and healthy living! You will be a winner in life when you Captain your life to success! – Patricia Bragg, Pioneer Health Crusader

---

Our habits, good or bad, are something we can control. – Dr. Edward Julius Stieglitz, author, "Geriatric Medicine" 1954

Seek and find the best for your body, mind and soul. – Patricia Bragg

Skin Problems and ACV Treatments

- **Cold sores and genital sores:** effectively relieve pain and discomfort caused by the herpes virus. Apply ACV directly to the affected areas and itching and burning will rapidly dissipate. Helps sores to heal more quickly.

- **Chicken pox:** caused by the herpes virus, can be relieved with straight ACV compresses. Apply ACV to the rash to help remove itchiness and limit spreading. Also try a warm bath with 1 cup ACV.

- **Psoriasis:** Gently apply to itching and burning areas. Also 2 cups ACV in warm bath also helps soothe itching.

- **Poison ivy and poison oak:** ACV relieves the itching and discomfort caused by these toxic plants. Mix equal parts of ACV and distilled water and spray on affected areas to stop pain, itching and ease redness and swelling. Keep ACV spray mixture in the refrigerator as chilled is more soothing.

- **Dry, itchy skin and hives:** Mix 2 Tbsps. cornstarch and enough ACV to form a paste. Apply on affected skin for 15 to 20 minutes. Wash off with lukewarm water.

- **Oily skin:** can be helped by the ACV drink (recipe on page 72) and the ACV Facial treatment twice a week (on page 39).

- **Varicose veins:** can be unsightly and painful, but applications of ACV can help shrink veins, along with taking Vitamin C, K and Rutin. Wrap an ACV-dampened cloth around needed areas morning and night, leaving on 15 minutes or longer, with your feet elevated up on a couch, against a wall or use a slant board. This brings more blood circulation to the legs. Then remove wrap, with your legs still up – start at the ankles to gently press over pooled veins to get blood back into circulation (see page 90 for more info on varicose veins).

I have the wisdom of my years and the youthfulness of The Bragg Healthy Lifestyle and I never act or feel my calendar years! I feel ageless! Why shouldn't you? Start living the Bragg Healthy Way today!
– Patricia Bragg

Age does not depend upon years, but upon lifestyle and health!

Apple Cider Vinegar for Sunburns

• **Windburn, sunburn and chapping (prevention):** coat the exposed skin with a mixture of 50/50 ACV and organic olive oil mixture. When in the weather elements, carry this mixture along in a small bottle.

• **For sunburn relief:** gently pat undiluted ACV on the skin or ACV compress. Leave ACV on to help prevent blistering and peeling. For all-over sunburns, pour a cup of ACV in warm bath water, then enjoy a healing soak. After soaking, gently dry your body, then pat ACV directly to needed areas. Wait 5 minutes, then pat on aloe vera gel.

"Organic Apple Cider Vinegar – the Best Burn Healer!"

We have used raw, organic apple cider vinegar for several years and love your wonderful book about it. We want to share with you something that we believe is one of the greatest benefits of organic apple cider vinegar brings to humanity (commercial vinegars don't have the same effect): organic apple cider vinegar, if splashed on a burn of any kind, stops the intense, continual pain instantly and permanently! It also prevents scarring and infection! We not only keep a bottle in our kitchen, we also keep bottles in our cars to use when people get burned from hot engines, radiators, etc. When traveling, we have helped burn victims from accidents in restaurant kitchens, cars, etc. We suggest everyone keep a bottle of apple cider vinegar nearby! Everyone who has tried it, has praised it! ACV is the best burn healer in the world, no matter how bad the burn! We thank you! – *Joel and N'omi Orr, Chesapeake, Virginia*

41

ACV for Lice, Insect Stings and Bites

• **Mosquito bites, insect bites, bee stings, scabies, head lice and jellyfish stings:** *ACV helps stop pain and itching and neutralizes their venom!* Use straight ACV on affected areas or diluted ACV compress as needed.

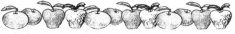

The human body has one ability not possessed by any machine – the body has the ability to repair and heal itself. – George W. Crile

ACV for Hemorrhoids and Rectal Itching

• **Hemorrhoids and rectal itching:** soak a cotton ball in ACV or witch hazel and gently press into area for relief.

ACV for Yeast and Fungus Problems

• **Yeast and fungus infections:** apply a 50/50 solution of ACV and distilled water topically on affected skin.

• **Athlete's Foot, Toenail Fungus, Jock Itch:** soak the affected area in a 50/50 mixture of ACV and lukewarm water for 10-30 minutes twice daily. Also try adding 2 Tbsps. of salt to water. After treatment, rinse, dry completely, and dust area with cornstarch.

• **Mouth thrush:** gargle every 3 hours with 1 tsp. ACV in half a glass of warm water. Also slowly drink warm apple cider vinegar drink morning and night, see recipe page 72.

• **Genital areas or diaper rash:** swab the affected area carefully 3 times daily with a solution of 1 Tbsp. apple cider vinegar to 1 quart of warm distilled water.

Treatments for all yeast and fungus infections should continue for at least 10 days or until symptoms dissipate.

ACV Bandages Stop Bleeding and Infection

• **For minor cuts and abrasions:** Healing is faster and there is less chance of infection if you swab areas daily with apple cider vinegar (perfect disinfectant and healer). ACV also helps stop bleeding by helping the blood to clot. Soak a cotton ball in ACV and press on abrasion until bleeding stops.

Studies show that apple cider vinegar soaked bandages quickly stop bleeding and prevent infection. The U.S. Army is currently testing these new bandages where urgency is so important to save lives! **Dad and I have had many miracle healings with vinegar for burns, cuts, bites, stings, infections, etc. as thousands of our readers have.**

Wake up and say, "Today I am going to be happier, healthier and wiser in my daily living because I am the captain of my life and in control to steer it for 100% healthy lifestyle living!" Fact: Happy people look younger, live longer, happier and have fewer health problems! – Patricia Bragg

Apple Cider Vinegar for Your Feet – Combatting Corns, Callouses and Warts

• **Corns and Callouses:** First soak the affected areas in warm water with ⅓ cup of ACV for 20 minutes. After soak, rub areas briskly with coarse towel, then gently use a pumice stone. Now apply full-strength ACV-soaked gauze bandage overnight, and in the morning prepare a fresh ACV soaked bandage for daytime use. These treatments help soften and dissolve corns and callouses. Check your shoes for comfort and fit. The wrong shoes are a main cause of corns, callouses, bunions and blisters. Give yourself weekly pedicures, massages and exercise your feet daily. Doing this while watching TV is ideal. Treat yourself to foot reflexology therapy (page 118). Walking barefoot on the sand, grass and at home is beneficial. Be good to your feet – they carry you through life! We kept famous foot Dr. William Scholl going strong, healthy and alert into his mid 80s!

• **Common Warts:** Use ACV treatment, *please use caution: do not rub warts, as this could spread them!* After soaking (see above), use ACV-soaked gauze, cover with waterproof tape, and keep gauze on overnight. In the morning, for daytime treatment, apply a castor oil-soaked gauze bandage. At night you can alternate ACV with vitamin E (pierce open an E capsule). Do this daily until completely gone. Combination of treatments work miracles! If your warts still become a problem, some doctors freeze them with liquid nitrogen. This method is fast, safe, easy and usually leaves no scars.

Remember – your feet are miracles in motion – be good to them!
– Paul C. Bragg, N.D., Ph.D., Health Crusader

Treatment of the feet to improve comfort and function will help favorably affect other parts of the body. – Elizabeth H. Roberts, DPM

People who habitually go barefoot have stronger, healthier feet than those who wear shoes. – Society for Barefoot Living • BareFooters.org

Progress is impossible without change, and those who cannot change their minds, cannot change anything. – George Bernard Shaw

ACV for Your Hair – Dandruff, Itching Scalp, Dry and Thinning Hair

The high acidity (organic malic acid) plus the powerful enzymes ("mother's" live chemicals) in ACV kill the bottle bacillus, a germ that can clog tiny openings and is responsible for many scalp and hair conditions such as dandruff, itching scalp, dry and thinning hair.

Every human hair has its own oil can. Scales and small dry crusts are formed, resulting in itching and dandruff. The oil-starved hairs either fall out or break off, causing hair thinning and baldness. ACV not only kills bottle bacillus, but stimulates the oil cans for healthier activity.

• **For dandruff:** put 2-3 Tbsps. of ACV in a cup – part hair in sections, and sponge ACV directly on your scalp. Wrap your head with a towel for 20 minutes. ACV helps restore scalp's proper acid/alkaline balance. Do before every shampoo.

• **For dry hair:** weekly apply organic olive oil to hair and ACV to scalp, then wrap with hot wet towel. Leave on for 30 minutes to 2 hours before shampooing.

• **To help stimulate hair growth and prevent hair loss**: Mix royal jelly capsule (*pierce open*) and 1 tsp. of apple cider vinegar. Pat on your bald areas, towel wrap, and leave on overnight. Many get great results.

Apple Cider Vinegar Hair Rinse Mixture for Shine and Body

Add 1/3 cup of apple cider vinegar to a quart of warm water. After shampooing/conditioning apply the vinegar rinse. Pour, squirt or spray the rinse onto wet hair. Massage into hair and scalp. Let sit for a couple of minutes to break up any residue. Rinse hair and dry as usual. Once your hair dries, it will not smell like vinegar! Pre-mix in handy plastic spray or squirt bottle and keep in shower to use.

ACV stimulates better blood circulation to hair follicles – something that is vital for encouraging hair growth and preventing hair loss. Furthermore, this blood carries essential nutrients to hair follicle cells, strengthening roots and promoting growth. – NaturalLivingIdeas.com

My father and I have shared The Bragg Healthy Lifestyle Blueprint with millions of people around the world at the Bragg Health and Fitness Crusades. I would now like to share it with you as part of the Apple Cider Vinegar Health Program.

With Blessings of Health, Peace, Joy and Love,

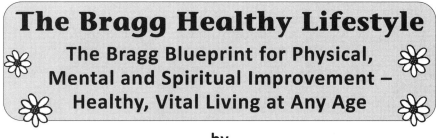

The Bragg Healthy Lifestyle
The Bragg Blueprint for Physical, Mental and Spiritual Improvement – Healthy, Vital Living at Any Age

by
Patricia Bragg
Life Extension Educator & Pioneer Health Crusader

Just think, in only 90 days you can build a new healthy bloodstream! Not a thick, sluggish, toxin-saturated bloodstream, but a rich, red bloodstream, healthy in all the vitamins, minerals and vital nutrients necessary for radiant and long lasting health. First and foremost, we must build the health content of our bloodstream. This is one of the great secrets of life: The more healthy nutrients in your bloodstream, the more oxygen is going to flood into your body, purifying its cells. Oxygen is the greatest natural stimulant. It stimulates, but doesn't depress. Unnatural stimulants stimulate, but there is an aftermath of depression! Tobacco, alcohol, coffee, tea, refined white sugar and flour and drugs (prescribed, street and over counter) have this bad effect on the body, but not oxygen – it's the invisible health staff of life!

So, in The Bragg Healthy Lifestyle we forever discard these harmful, destructive stimulants! You are going to be strong and never allow these to enter your body again! You are going to rely on the many wonderful, natural stimulants to create a more healthy body and vital force.

Man's days shall be to 120 years. – Genesis 6:3

First, you are now going to start breathing deeper and slower, as it's important for super energy! Then you are going to eat organic, live foods, such as fresh salads, fruits, vegetables and fresh blended or squeezed juices, that build up your blood, health and energy.

Before you eat or drink anything, I want you to ask yourself this important question, "Is this going to build a healthy bloodstream or destroy it?" Be on the alert to protect your precious river of life – your bloodstream! **When it demands liquids, give it the best – purified distilled water and live-food juices, as fresh organic fruit and vegetable juices.** Buy a blender – *Nutri-Bullet* or a juicer. Every day fortify your blood with fresh orange, grapefruit and fruit and carrot and green juices or combine juices such as celery, tomato, beet and parsley or see page 109. Four of the best juices to add to vegetable juices are raw spinach, kale, cabbage and watercress. For a taste delight, add juice of 1 to 2 garlic buds (wrap in veg leaf to juice). Garlic is an excellent purifier and heart protector.

Do not consume too much of these powerful, live-food juices. One to two pints a day is more than enough! Some people get a juicer and overdo it. Overloading your body with juices can upset your delicate blood-sugar balance. Eating the whole fruit is still the best! Just because something is good for you doesn't mean that a lot of it is. As with all things in life, moderation of your food intake is best for building Health Vitality Supreme!

Imagine: In just 11 months you will have an absolutely "new you!" The billions of soft cells that make up your eyes, nose, skin, hands and feet, as well as all the vital organs of your body, will be renewed! You do not need to submit to the huge risk of heart, kidney or any other dangerous transplant operations!

You have within your power, through the food you eat, the liquid you drink and the air you breathe, the ability to build a fresh, vital body from the top of your head to the tip of your toes! What you eat and drink today will be walking and talking tomorrow! How wonderful our Creator has been to us, to give us the miracle power every 90 days to build a new bloodstream and every 11 months, an amazing healthier body!

Stop Dying – Start Healthy Living Now!
The Bible tells us that . . .
The kingdom of Heaven is within us.

We thoroughly believe this statement! We can make this body we live in either a kingdom of heaven on Earth or we can make it a torture chamber. It's all up to you! After childhood, the kind of body you live in is strictly up to you! We cannot live your life for you! Nor can anyone else! You are a mature adult, and you must face the realities of life. **I am sure you have the willpower and desire to follow The Bragg Healthy Lifestyle, so start now on the Royal Road to Higher Health – start today!**

This is the Bragg Master Blueprint to greater physical perfection because it works with the Laws of God and Mother Nature, and they make no compromises! You either follow them or they break you! You can't break a Natural Law or God's Law, for it will break you in time!

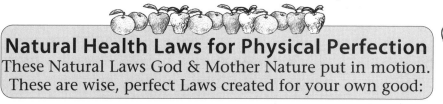

Natural Health Laws for Physical Perfection 47
These Natural Laws God & Mother Nature put in motion.
These are wise, perfect Laws created for your own good:

- *You must eat natural foods for super health (page 57).*
- *You must breathe deeply of pure air (page 77).*
- *You must exercise and keep good posture (page 81 and 87).*
- *You must give your body pure, safe, clean water (page 93).*
- *You must give your body gentle sunshine (page 99).*
- *You must rest – don't overwork or burden your body; this leads to stress and nerve depletion (page 101).*
- *You must keep the body clean inside by fasting (page 105).*
- *You must live by divine intelligence and wisdom (page 111).*

The human body is a miracle, give it the best. Within us is the inherent potential to become perfect! It is the intent of our Creator for us to have a physically perfect, healthy, happy and peaceful long life! – Genesis 6:3

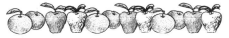

No act of kindness, no matter how small, is never wasted. – Aesop, 600 B.C.

Enjoy Mother Nature's and God's Foods

When we are not physically perfect, we are out of harmony with the Creator's design, and therefore out of harmony with God's intent, will and law (3 John 2). In simpler words, we are, in our unhealthy living habits, opposing the will of God and Mother Earth. So, you see that to reach physical perfection, we must live correctly on all four important planes: the physical, the mental, the emotional and the spiritual. By living on the physical plane correctly, we can then reach a higher mental, emotional and spiritual state for healthy perfection.

If you eat Mother Nature's Foods and build a healthy, clean bloodstream, you are going to be keener mentally! The wonderful part of living by this blueprint is that we find a new calmness coming over us. You'll experience a new feeling of confidence, peace, joy and serenity! When every cell, organ and body part is functioning perfectly, the body becomes more perfect physically, mentally, emotionally and spiritually. **What complete satisfaction you will feel when you live The Bragg Healthy Lifestyle and reap the great rewards of a healthier, happier, stronger and more fulfilled life!**

Your degree of physical perfection is the measure of your efforts in cooperating by daily partaking of proper foods, exercise, deep breathing and youthful thinking. This is your Creator's health design and intent so that you can become strong and remain physically healthy, youthful, active and of service, regardless of your age! Four exemplary long lives of devoted service we admire: Albert Einstein, Gandhi, Albert Schweitzer and Mother Teresa.

Spread love everywhere. Be the living expression of God's kindness – kindness in your face, kindness in your eyes, kindness in your smiles, kindness in your warm greetings. – Mother Teresa

Fruits and vegetables bear closest relation to light. The sun pours a continuous flood of light into them to furnish us the healthiest and best food a human being requires for sustenance of mind, body and life. – Louisa May Alcott, author of novel, "Little Women" 1832-1888

Organic fruits & vegetables are filled with life for health of mind & body!

THE BRAGG HEALTHY LIFESTYLE
Promotes Super Health and Longevity

The Bragg Healthy Lifestyle consists of eating a diet of 60% to 70% fresh, live, organically grown foods; raw vegetables, salads, fresh fruits and juices; sprouts, raw seeds and raw nuts; all-natural 100% whole-grain breads, pastas, cereals and nutritious beans and legumes. These are the no cholesterol, no fat, no salt, "live foods" which combine to make up the body fuel that creates healthy, lively people that want to exercise and be fit. This healthy diet also creates energy. This is the reason people become revitalized and reborn into a fresh new life filled with joy, health, vitality, youthfulness and longevity! **There are millions of healthy Bragg followers around the world proving The Bragg Healthy Lifestyle works miracles!**

If you want more health, energy and a longer life, you will have to plan, plot and start creating, becoming and shaping your life! Look ahead. Have firm plans for living your life. Actually envision your future. You may change those plans and visions, but have them you must! Your creative force deep within you must reach out toward a brighter future if you want to become one with the healthy flow for an exciting, fulfilling life! Your entire mind and being will be super energized in the process to go for your future goals and dreams.

 49

It's Never Too Late For You
to Seek and Build Radiant Health!

The Creator gave us a brain for intelligence and reasoning power to take control of our body! But flesh is dumb! You can stuff anything in your stomach and almost get away with it until the day of reckoning arrives! Most young people live this way, because they falsely believe they are totally indestructible! But what a sad lesson they learn after 30 or 40 years of wrong living! The infirmities and the aches and pains creep into their bodies, making life miserable and proving to them that their dream of indestructibility was a myth and a lie!

Live by a wise reasoning mind, rather than by the senses of the body. The dumb senses are constantly enticing you to do the very things that destroy your miracle body. Look around you at the sad, broken-down human sights you see.

Whatsoever a man soweth, he shall also reap. – The Bible

We should know and observe the fact everything in the universe is always governed by definite wise laws. If we understand and follow these universal health laws we will sow seeds of constructive, healthy living!

Make every day a healthy day and each day you will improve! You will feel new strength and energy flooding into your body! The feelings you will experience when you live 100% The Bragg Healthy Lifestyle are indescribable! What an incredibly powerful and joyful feeling it is to be fully alive and vigorous, with unlimited energy and powerful nerve force. An amazing example, the life of ageless, energy-filled Jack LaLanne – page 86.

Busy people often make excuses to continue living their current unhealthy lifestyle. They will tell you they are too old to begin The Bragg Healthy Lifestyle Program. Age has no force, nor is it toxic! Time is just a measure.

Millions Suffer from Premature Ageing

There are millions in their 30s, 40s and 50s who are, sad to say, prematurely old biologically. Yet there are many in their 70s, 80s and 90s who are biologically youthful, active, healthy and happy! **The second half of life is best!**

In our opinion, if you are experiencing premature ageing, you are suffering from a highly toxic condition and from unnecessary nutritional deficiencies. These are the main causes of most human troubles. The Bragg Healthy Lifestyle will show you how to banish these vicious enemies. From this minute on, stop living by calendar years! Just forget your birthdays, as we do. All of us are reborn every second of the day as new body cells are being constantly created.

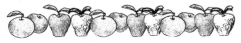

Time waits for no one, treasure and protect every moment you have!

Cease this talk of getting old! From this minute on, you will have no age except your biological age and this you are going to control. **Every day say to yourself . . .**

I Will Stay Healthy, Youthful, Active and Happy!

Say it repeatedly, burn it deeply into your mind and it will sparkle all your days for your entire long happy life!

Most people have a dreadful fear of getting old. They picture themselves half blind, hearing impaired, with teeth and hair gone, energy and vitality spent or senile. They see themselves as a burden to their family and friends. They envision themselves in a nursing home alone, forgotten, maybe with Alzheimer's disease.

Despite the fear of old age and the train of ailments that go with it, you can prevent this human tragedy! You can skip this terrible period by changing how you live from this day forward! Today is the day to prepare against becoming senile and decrepit! That's why I urge you to **follow the Wise Laws of God and Mother Nature. You will grow younger as you live longer! That is what this Bragg Health Program is all about: The preservation of your precious vital health for a long, fulfilled life!**

51

The Body Has the Seed of Eternal Life

Health, like freedom and peace, lasts as long as we exert ourselves to maintain it. You must make your choice! It's almost exclusively in your hands whether you enjoy a healthy, vigorous life to a ripe old age or live out a half-alive, non-energetic existence with premature breakdown of health. It has been proven by some of the greatest scientific minds that there are no special diseases of old age. A person should not die simply because they live to 60, 70, 80 or 90 years of age, because calendar age is not toxic. People create their toxins by their lifestyle of eating and living habits.

Many people die of some fatal condition that they have built into their bodies by incorrect living or by violating the natural laws that govern the physical body.

A strong body and a bright, happy, serene countenance can only result from thoughts of joy, goodwill and serenity into the mind and heart.
– James Allen, inspirational author, "As A Man Thinketh" – 1903

The two great enemies of life are toxic poisons (found in some foods, air, water and soil) and the nutritional deficiencies caused by an unhealthy diet. The best prevention of sickness is to eat vital, healthy foods (organic is best and safer), especially those high in potassium. These provide the body with correct, life-giving nourishment.

Every 90 days a new bloodstream, the river of life, is built in the body by the foods you eat, the liquids you drink and the air you breathe! From your bloodstream the body's cells are made, nourished and maintained. Every 11 months we have a new set of billions of miraculous body cells, and every two years we have an entirely new set of bones and hard tissues. There is no reason to get old because the body is constantly cleansing and renewing its cells to keep your precious miracle human temple healthy for a long, fulfilled, happy life!

Wise Prevention Helps Keep You Healthy, Youthful and Vigorous!

Lengthening life by special treatment for chronic miseries often means merely adding years of ill health and misery to a person's life. This is often called *the living death*. Who wants to extend life just to suffer? We say, the healer's function is to prevent sickness and disease. No person is able to heal you! Only you can heal yourself! **In order to be healthy it's essential to learn how to live healthy in order to be healthy always. They say –**

An ounce of prevention is worth a ton of cure!

My father and I always stressed to our readers that prevention is always healthiest, best and is priceless!

Diet for Health and Youthfulness – Your diet should be composed of 60% – 70% raw organic fruits, prunes, salads and raw or steamed, baked, or wokked veggies. Conditions such as stomach upsets, miseries and constipation that occur in children and adults, can then be avoided (pages 20-21). Output should equal intake. You should have a bowel movement soon upon arising in morning and after meals.

The greatest enemy of health is constipation, but this can be eliminated by a diet that gives you sufficient bulk, moisture, lubrication and vigorous exercise of the entire abdominal cavity (see pages 20-21 and 81). In remote parts of the world, where we traveled beyond influences of so-called modern civilization, mankind indulges in the normal habit of defecation soon after meals. Best to train yourself to have bowel movements after arising and after meals. Children can be taught this important healthy habit from infancy. Living The Bragg Healthy Lifestyle faithfully, constipation soon vanishes!

Good Elimination is Vital to Health

Studies reveal the presence of toxic poisons in cases of constipation. When these toxins are absorbed into the general circulation, the liver "your detoxifying organ" is unable to cope with them. These toxins are then thrown back into the body to cause degenerative diseases, toxemia, cancer, premature ageing, sickness and lack of energy.

Your lifestyle and diet play a vital role in the maintenance of your health, good elimination and the prevention of disease. Research shows that diets composed of refined white flour and sugar; preserved meats, such as hot dogs and luncheon meats; white rice; coffee, tea, cola drinks and all alcohol; overcooked vegetables; and high fat, sugared, salted, and processed foods create serious health problems, especially in the colon and intestinal tract, heart and respiratory areas. **It's wise to never eat refined, processed, embalmed and dead, unhealthy foods!!!**

The Body is Self-Cleansing, Self-Healing and Self-Repairing

It's our duty if we want vibrant, glorious health, to do all we can to make the body work efficiently to maintain vital, super health. Not only is a healthy diet necessary, but so are good sleeping habits, outdoor physical activity, full, deep breathing and a serene, peaceful mind! We cannot live by bread alone. We must have spiritual food. Please strive for a perfect healthy balance: physical, mental, emotional and spiritual well-being!

Your Energy is Your Body's Spark Plug

Your energy comes from the spark of life, which is maintained by the atomic energy contained within every single cell of the human body. It embodies electrons, protons and neutrons. They are constantly discharging their ionic compounds as energy is expended in work or play, whether mental or physical, in accordance with natural laws. This energy loss must be replaced. Every cell in your body is like a battery that, when run down, must be recharged! Primarily, this is done through the intake of food, proper breathing, rest and exercise which help recharge your billions of cells!

Now, **there are two kinds of food: The first is in a low rate of health vibration,** sadly, like fast junk foods we mentioned: the processed, chemicalized, dead foods, as in refined white flour and sugars, etc. It's impossible to have a youthful, dynamic body when, year after year, you feed it food and drinks with a low rate of vibration.

54

Healthy Foods Give High Health Vibrations They Contain Life-Giving Substances

When you eat only foods that are in a high health vibration, your body performs and operates by God's Universal Law and becomes a miracle self-starting, self-governing, self-generating instrument! We want you to live by Mother Nature's and God's Laws so your body will be a miracle working instrument for a long life! If you have the desire to retain vitality, energy and enthusiasm of youth and the desire to turn back the clock of Father Time – you can start now! If your body is bent, eyes are dimmed and gait is halting when you should be buoyant with the spirit of youthfulness, then please start now. We say:

❀ *"There is but one way to live and that is* ❀
Mother Nature's and God's Healthy Way!"

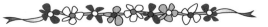

With every new day comes new strength and new thoughts.
– Eleanor Roosevelt, First Lady, U.S. President, Franklin D. Roosevelt

You are what you Eat, Drink, Breathe, Think, Say and Do! – Patricia Bragg

The Bragg Healthy Lifestyle Program consists only of **foods** in a **high rate of health vibration.** Many have the preconceived idea that animal protein is the highest rate of food. While protein is an important nutrient to the body, healthier vegetarian protein is best! Organic fresh fruits and vegetables have high health vibrations. Fruit produces blood sugar, which helps to feed the nerves of the body. Fruit has a two fold purpose in the body. First, it's rich in blood sugar; second, it's also an important detoxifier and destroyer of harmful toxins.

Body Cleansing & Healthy Transition Diet

People who have been living on a diet high in animal proteins, fats, salt, starches and refined sugars can't immediately include a large amount of fresh fruits and vegetables in their diet. It's best to slowly ease into The Bragg Healthy Lifestyle to allow the body to cleanse itself gently.

Everyone who wants to live a healthy life must thoroughly understand just what is going on in their body chemistry! Fresh, organic, raw fruits and vegetables help flush toxins out. The body can't be rushed. It takes the average person a long time to saturate the body with toxic poisons. Now it's going to take time to flush this debris out with this transition diet!

55

The more organic raw fruits and raw vegetables that you condition yourself to handle, the more cleansed your body will become! So, recognize these foods, which are in the highest rate of healthy vibration. But please, also respect their cleansing and detoxifying action!

> **We often eat 100% raw meals of fruits, veggies or salads for a few days, but usually our meals are 60% -70% raw.**

Breakfast: Fresh, raw juice (orange, grapefruit, carrot, celery, garlic, spinach, etc.) or raw fruit (in season, melon, apricot, berry, peach, nectarine) or the nutritious, delicious Bragg Energy Smoothie, see recipe on page 72.

There is truth in the saying that man becomes what he eats. – Gandhi

Lunch: Large variety salad with fresh greens, vegetables, sprouts and a few raw nuts or seeds (sunflower, pinenuts, pumpkin, almonds, pecans, walnuts, etc.), recipe on page 73.

Dinner: Variety salad, followed by two steamed, baked or stir fried in a wok fresh organic vegetables and one of following: beans, lentils, organic brown rice, whole grain pasta, baked or steamed potatoes.

Remember to get your daily ACV into your diet with the ACV drink and sprinkle olive oil over steamed greens, cauliflower, squash, broccoli, cabbage, stringbeans, etc.

People are told they must start the day with a big breakfast, to give them great energy in the morning hours. So, they gorge themselves on processed cereal with milk and sugar; ham and eggs; or bacon and eggs; stacks of hot cakes or buttered toast and jelly. All of this is washed down with coffee, milk or cocoa. You will note that there are no fresh fruits at this meal. Only a person doing the most strenuous physical labor could possibly burn up a meal like this, and we doubt that even they could. All the vital energy of the body will be needed to digest these heavy animal proteins and fats, refined starch and white sugar breakfasts! All too often, they lie in the stomach like a ton of bricks and have to be dynamited out! Now you know why there is so much indigestion, constipation, colon cancer and why laxatives are some of the biggest sellers in drugstores!

How can a big meal like this give a person strength for their morning duties? The truth is, it can't! This is how parents and, consequently, their children are brainwashed by big food interests who sell all their commercial, sugared, unhealthy, worthless foods! You must change your ideas about food! **Learn to eat in moderation. It's important not to overfuel and store excess pounds on your body! If you overfeed your body, you clog it up! A diet of healthy, organic, raw and cooked foods with a high vibration rate will help keep your insides clean and you healthier!**

The human body is its own best medicine. The most successful prescriptions are those filled by the body itself.
– Norman Cousins, author, "Anatomy of An Illness"

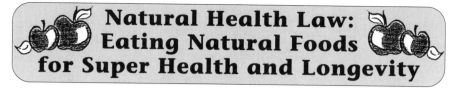

Natural Health Law:
Eating Natural Foods
for Super Health and Longevity

Bad Nutrition is #1 Cause of Sickness

*"Diet-related diseases account
for 68% of all deaths."*
– Dr. C. Everett Koop

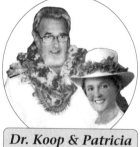

Dr. Koop & Patricia
Hawaii Health Conference

America's former top Surgeon General and our friend, said this in his famous 1988 landmark report on nutrition and health in America. People don't die of infectious conditions as such, but of malnutrition that allows the germs to get a foothold in sickly bodies. Also, bad nutrition is usually the cause of non-infectious, fatal or degenerative conditions. When the body has its full nutrition quota of vitamins and minerals, including potassium, it's almost impossible for germs to get a foothold in a healthy, powerful bloodstream and tissues!

57

Millions Suffer from Malnutrition

"Mal" means bad. As a consequence of not getting natural, healthy, balanced diets, millions worldwide suffer from many forms of subclinical malnutrition. This means many people, due to vitamin and mineral deficiencies, feel unwell most of the time! They lack vim, vigor and "Go Power" and feel tired. Their daily food intake and the commercial vinegars they use don't provide sufficient vitamins and minerals, nor the potassium their bodies require. They lack vital power and feel exhausted. This is the reason people turn to stimulants like coffee, colas, alcohol, cigarettes and over-the-counter "fix-all" drugs. After these stimulants' effects wear off, they feel terrible. They just exist, and are not living happy, healthy lives!

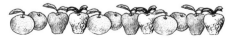

*"Paul Bragg did more for the Health of America than any one
person I know of." – Former US Surgeon General, C. Everett Koop*

Vegetarians Are Healthier and Live Longer

Most uninformed nutritionists call meat the #1 source of protein. Those proteins coming from the vegetable kingdom are referred to as the #2 proteins (see page 69). This is a sad and terrible mistake! It should be the other way around! In this day and age, almost all meat is laden with herbicides, fungicides, pesticides and other chemicals that are sprayed on or poured into the feed which these animals consume! They are also pumped full of hormones, antibiotics, growth stimulators and toxic drugs to fatten them up and keep them from dying from the unhealthy conditions they live in! Beware of animal products!

Start Eating Healthy Foods For Super Energy

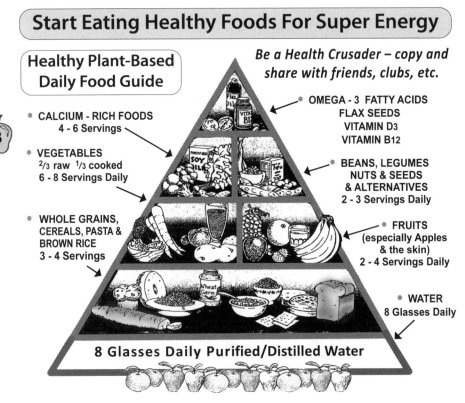

Healthy Plant-Based Daily Food Guide

Be a Health Crusader – copy and share with friends, clubs, etc.

58

- CALCIUM - RICH FOODS
  4 - 6 Servings

- VEGETABLES
  2/3 raw 1/3 cooked
  6 - 8 Servings Daily

- WHOLE GRAINS, CEREALS, PASTA & BROWN RICE
  3 - 4 Servings

- OMEGA - 3 FATTY ACIDS
  FLAX SEEDS
  VITAMIN D3
  VITAMIN B12

- BEANS, LEGUMES
  NUTS & SEEDS
  & ALTERNATIVES
  2 - 3 Servings Daily

- FRUITS
  (especially Apples & the skin)
  2 - 4 Servings Daily

- WATER
  8 Glasses Daily

8 Glasses Daily Purified/Distilled Water

The *Healthy Plant-Based Daily Food Guide Pyramid* illustration above, represents an ideal way of eating for achieving optimal nutrition, health and longevity! You will notice that this Food Guide Pyramid is based on healthy organic plant-based foods, with emphasis on fruits, vegetables, whole grains, vegetable protein foods, non-dairy calcium foods, raw nuts, seeds and purified water. This is the best diet for building a healthy nervous system, disease prevention and to enjoy longevity. *Eating a diet based on these dietary guidelines will help get the nutrients you need for optimal health:*

PURIFIED WATER: The pyramid's foundation. We recommend drinking *pure distilled water* as it is the best type of water for the body. However other clean waters like reverse osmosis or pure spring are good. Drink at least eight – 8 oz glasses of pure water daily and even more if your lifestyle (sports, work, etc.) requires it. Read our *Water – The Shocking Truth.*

WHOLE GRAINS: Whole grains are next pyramid level. **Avoid all GMO process, refined grain products** and eat only unrefined, organic whole grain bread and cereals. Grains such as whole wheat, brown rice, oats, millet, quinoa, and 100% whole grain breads and cereals are best. One serving of whole grains is equal to 1 slice whole grain bread, 1 ounce ready-to-eat whole grain cereal, 1 cup cooked whole grains such as brown rice, oatmeal or other grains, 1 cup whole wheat, rice, pasta or noodles, and 1 ounce other whole grain products. *We recommend eating 3-4 servings whole grains a day.* This is because it is challenging to find truly GMO-free wheat in America. Many people of all ages discover they are gluten-sensitive. The wheat of today is not the wheat our grandparents consumed (see pages 62-63). Gluten-free grains such as rice, buckwheat and quinoa are easier to digest and create less mucus as well.

VEGETABLES: We recommend eating as many of your vegetables organic and raw (uncooked, in salads, juices, smoothies, etc.) as possible! When cooking vegetables, do not overcook them. Steaming or lightly stir-frying is best. **The more colorful rainbow of vegetables you eat, the better they are for your health as they contain more valuable nutrients and healthy phytochemicals (page 71).** Eat a wide variety of organic vegetables daily. One vegetable serving is equal to 1 cup cooked vegetables or 1 cup raw uncooked vegetables, 1 cup salad, 3/4 cup vegetable juice. *We recommend 6-8 or more vegetable servings daily.*

Enjoy healthy, organic foods for their wonderful abundance of life energy

FRUITS: Like vegetables, the more colorful the fruits the more healthy for you! Enjoy organic fruits as often as possible! One serving of fruit is equal to 1 medium apple, banana, orange, pear or other fruit, 1/2 cup fruit, 1/2 cup of fruit juice or 1/4 cup dried fruit. *We recommend eating 2-4 servings or more of organic fruits daily.*

CALCIUM FOODS: Are plant-derived calcium-rich foods. Plant sources of calcium are healthier than dairy products because they don't contain saturated fats or cholesterol. Health calcium-rich foods are: soymilk, tofu, broccoli and green leafy vegetables. Serving sizes of plant-derived calcium-rich foods include: 1 cup soymilk, 1/2 cup tofu, 1/3 cup almonds, 1 cup cooked or 2 cups of high calcium raw greens (kale, collards, broccoli, bok choy or other Chinese greens), 1 cup of calcium-rich beans (e.g. soy, white, navy, Great Northern), 1/2 cup seaweed, 1 tablespoon blackstrap molasses, 5 or more figs. *We recommend having 4-6 servings of healthy non-dairy sources of calcium rich foods daily.*

BEANS & LEGUMES: Are healthy protein foods. Vegetable protein foods are more optimal compared to animal protein foods (plant-based protein chart, see page 69). Vegetable proteins do not contain artery clogging saturated fats and cholesterol found in animal foods. They also contain protective factors to prevent heart disease, cancer and diabetes. Vegetable proteins provide the body with essential amino acids that it requires. One serving of vegetable protein foods include: 1 cup cooked legumes (beans, lentils, dried peas), 1/2 cup firm tofu or tempeh, 1 serving of "veggie meat," 3 tablespoons nut or seed butter, 1 cup soy, almond or rice milk. *We recommend 2-3 or more vegetable protein servings daily.*

ESSENTIAL NUTRIENTS: are essential and healthy fats, like Omega-3's, vitamin D3 and minerals. Servings of healthy fats include: 1 tsp. of flaxseed oil, 1 Tbsp. of organic extra virgin olive oil, 3 tsps. of raw walnuts or pumpkin seeds. Other healthy essential nutrients include: ground flaxseeds or chia seeds and nutritional B-Complex supplements that provide vitamin B12. Do provide your body with nutritional supplements your body requires for optimal health and longevity!

Internal Cleanliness is the Secret of Health

What you want to strive for is a clean, toxicless body! Gradually include more organic fresh raw fruits and raw vegetables in your diet. Have fresh fruits in the morning and a large raw, combination vegetable salad at noon. If you like, you may have some fresh fruit for dessert. Eat a yellow vegetable, such as a yam, sweet potato, yellow squash or carrots, and a green vegetable every day. Cook vegetables by baking, steaming or stir-frying them. Remember to save some raw vegetables for your cleansing Raw Organic Vegetable Health Salad (recipe on page 73).

With your main meal you may have and want a more concentrated form of protein. Our favorite and healthiest proteins are vegetarian! If you eat animal or sea food proteins, have (hormone-free) not over 2 times a week. Your diet should include raw nuts and seeds: almonds, cashews, peanuts, pecans, pine nuts, pumpkins, sesame, sunflower, walnuts and avocados. Enjoy beans, brown rice and legumes, soybeans and tofu as often as desired. By having a variety of natural foods you will enjoy a balanced healthier diet and a long, healthier life! 61

You may use natural, cold or expeller pressed oils such as: olive, flax, soy, safflower, sunflower and sesame. Read labels carefully before buying! We put organic extra virgin, cold pressed olive oil over our baked potatoes, instead of salt-free butter. It's also perfect over brown rice, lentils, beans and vegetables. We never use table salt – it should have no place in your diet! This kind of salt is an inorganic substance that causes health problems. Organic sodium found naturally in "live" foods is best. (Himalayan Salt is okay.) Read labels, don't buy products that add iodized salt!

The best way to eat potatoes is baked. We use a fast baking method. Thoroughly scrub potato (either white, yam or sweet). Don't wrap or oil it. Bake in 450°F oven for 25 minutes. Do eat the skin, too! Baked this way, it's crunchy and delicious. We don't believe in microwaves that destroy food cells, as irradiation also does! (See page 63.) A convection oven is safer and almost as fast as microwave and can be placed on kitchen counter-top.

Avocado is Mother Nature's miracle food: The avocado tree is strong and it requires no spraying with poisonous chemicals. The avocado has a perfect balance of life-giving nutrients (potassium, folic acid, fiber, niacin, B6, protein, etc.). It's unsaturated fat helps lower LDL "bad" cholesterol. We eat avocados from our Santa Barbara Farm three times weekly. Mash the avocado, add fresh minced garlic, salsa, lime juice, and organic olive oil. Dip slices of tomato, celery, carrot, turnip, cabbage, red onion, cucumber, bell pepper and lettuce leaves into this "guacamole" for a delicious healthy lunch.

Beware: Why "Modern" Wheat is Bad for You

Modern wheat isn't really wheat at all and is a "perfect, chronic poison", according to Dr. William Davis, a Cardiologist, author and leading expert on wheat, the world's most popular grain. *Dr. Davis explains that the wheat we eat today (even though it may say 100% whole wheat), isn't the wheat your ancestors had, it's an 18" tall plant created by genetic research in the 60's and 70's. There's a new protein in this type of wheat called Gliadin, which is an opiate. Gliadin binds into opiate receptors in brain and in most people stimulates appetite – they consume 440 more calories per day, 365 days per year.

Modern wheat is responsible for eight out of ten people's health problems. Researchers have found that once wheat is removed from their diet, their illnesses disappeared within three to six months. People who turn away from wheat have dropped substantial weight. Even diabetics benefit. People with arthritis have dramatic relief. Along with less acid reflux; leg swelling; irritable bowel syndrome, as well as depression.

So why is wheat bad? Wheat is one of the oldest known grains. When grown in organic, fertile soil, non-GMO whole wheat is rich in vitamins E and B complex, many minerals, including calcium and iron, as well as omega-3 fatty acids.

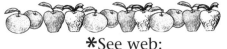

*See web:
IntentionalWellnessInc.com/nutrition/wheat-is-bad-for-you

Unfortunately, the modern version of wheat is a far cry from the ancient plant. As with other commercially grown grains, scientists began cross-breeding wheat plants to arrive at new varieties that are hardier, shorter, and yield more. In fact, the newer, high-yield hybridized wheat we've been eating since the 1980's has been selectively bred to produce high gluten grains that seem to trigger inflammatory responses in our body, causing more problems than ever! Among the diseases attributed to the consumption of wheat is Celiac disease.

Dr. Davis says, "that there is no nutrient deficiency that develops when eliminating wheat from your diet. Replace wheat with organic healthy foods like vegetables; nuts, avocados. Try eliminating grains, that's when you will see transformations in your health."

Warning! – Avoid All Microwaved Foods Beware – They Are Unhealthy!

In the past 40 years (health destroying) microwaves have practically replaced traditional methods of cooking, especially with on-the-go people of today's world. But how much do you really know about them? Are they no more than timesaving machines for cooking? A Swiss Study found that food which is microwaved is not the food it was before! The microwave radiation deforms and destroys the molecular structure of the food – creating radiolytic compounds! When microwaved food is eaten, abnormal changes then occur in your blood and immune systems! These include a decrease in hemoglobin and white blood cell counts and increase in cholesterol levels! An article in *Pediatrics Journal* warns microwaving human milk damages the anti-infective properties it usually gives to a mother's baby. Research done at University of Warwick in Great Britain warned that microwave radiation damaged the vital electromagnetic activity of human life vibrations. Over 20 years ago Russia established wise microwave radiation limits more stringent than United States and Great Britain! **Beware please don't use microwaves!!**

You can be a sewage system when eating unhealthy, highly processed foods. Remember, live organic foods produce healthy, living, live people!

Avoid Refined, Processed, Unhealthy Foods!

Eliminate refined, white flour products and white sugar products entirely. Eat no mushy, dead, refined cereals or those dry sugared cereals, they are unhealthy despite some being enriched with chemically produced vitamins and minerals. (Health Stores carry natural organic whole-grains cereals, granola, breads, rolls, pastas, even pastries.)

Avoid these foods: Fried, salted, refined, preserved and chemicalized foods; coffee, black and green (caffeine) teas, cola, soft drinks, sugared drinks and alcohol drinks; overcooked, over-salted vegetables and salted, creamed and white flour-thickened soups. Please read page 66 for a complete foods-to-avoid list for alert wise health buying.

You now know the foods to avoid: Refined, unhealthy foods high in fat, salt and sugar; meat and dairy products; sugared foods and beverages, chemicalized water and foods.

You now know the foods you can eat: Fresh fruits (organically grown is always best to buy or grow yourself); fresh juices; raw salads; fresh vegetables – raw, steam, bake or wok; vegetable proteins, beans, legumes, tofu, raw nuts, seeds, etc. If you really want animal and fish proteins, limit to twice weekly. Occasionally, eat nothing but fresh fruits, raw vegetables and sprouts for 1 or 2 days a week. Remember, vegetarians are healthiest among Americans! Research proves this! See web: *ornish.com*

Use your imagination to plan enjoyable, live food meals that are powerful for super health! Keep meals simple! Avoid eating too many food mixtures. Don't overeat! Be moderate in all things for the best of health! Eat only when you are really hungry, not because it is mealtime. Earn your food by activity, vigorous exercise and deep breathing. You will see how much more you really enjoy your food when you deserve and earn it!

64

There's no substitute for a healthy diet of organic fruits, vegetables, grains and legumes. Vitamin deficiency usually occurs only after many weeks or months of intake below recommended daily levels.
– "The Complete Guide to Natural Healing" by Tom Monte

Stevia – The Natural Herbal Sweetener

Stevia is an herb native to South America. It's widely grown for its sweet leaves. In its unprocessed form it's 30 times sweeter than sugar. It is low in carbohydrates. Stevia or monk fruit show promise for treating conditions such as obesity and high blood pressure. They don't affect blood sugar and even enhance glucose tolerance. Both make a safe, delicious, health sweetener for diabetics. Children can use them without concerns as they do not cause cavities.

Beware of Deadly Aspartame and Other Sugar Substitutes

Although its name sounds "tame," this deadly neurotoxin is anything but! Aspartame is an artificial sweetener (over 200 times sweeter than sugar) made by Monsanto Corporation and marketed as "NutraSweet," "Equal," "Spoonful," and countless other trade names. Although aspartame is added to over 9,000 food products, it is not fit for human consumption! This toxic poison changes into formaldehyde in the body and has been linked to migraines, seizures, vision loss and symptoms relating to lupus, Parkinson's Disease, Multiple Sclerosis and other health destroying conditions (even Gulf War Syndrome). For more info on this toxic killer – this crime against our health, check webs: *aspartame.mercola.com* and *holisticmed.com/aspartame.*

65

Organic natural foods are the greatest source for staying healthy!
– Patricia Bragg, Pioneer Health Crusader

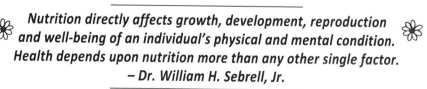

Seek and choose whole foods, organic fruits, vegetables and organic whole grain cereals, breads, etc. rather than commercial, canned, refined white flour, sugar products and other highly processed goods in the center aisles.

Nutrition directly affects growth, development, reproduction and well-being of an individual's physical and mental condition. Health depends upon nutrition more than any other single factor.
– Dr. William H. Sebrell, Jr.

Organic vegetables are a key to staying healthy. They are full of fiber and antioxidants which trap the free-radical molecules that can cause cancer.
– Connie Mobley, Ph.D., R.D., University of Texas Health Sciences Center

Avoid These Processed, Refined, Harmful Foods:

Once you realize the harm caused to your body by unhealthy refined, chemicalized, deficient foods, you'll want to eliminate "killer" foods:

- **Refined sugar / artificial sweeteners** (toxic aspartame) or their products such as jams, jellies, preserves, marmalades, yogurts, ice cream, sherbets, Jello, cake, candy, cookies, all chewing gum, colas and diet drinks, pies, pastries, and all sugared fruit juices and fruits canned in sugar syrup. (Health Stores have delicious healthy replacements, such as Stevia, raw honey, 100% maple syrup, and agave nectar, so seek and buy the best).

- **White flour products** such as white bread, wheat-white bread, enriched flours, rye bread that has white flour in it, dumplings, biscuits, buns, gravy, pasta, pancakes, waffles, soda crackers, pizza, ravioli, pies, pastries, cakes, cookies, prepared and commercial puddings and ready-mix bakery products. Most are made with dangerous (oxy-cholesterol) powdered milk and powdered eggs. (Health Stores have a variety of 100% non-GMO whole grain organic products, breads, chips, crackers, pastas, desserts).

- **Salted foods**, such as pretzels, corn chips, potato chips, crackers and nuts.

- **Refined white rice** and pearl barley. • **Fried fast foods.** • **Indian ghee.**

- **Refined dry processed cereals** that are sugared, such as cornflakes, etc.

- **Foods that contain Olestra**, palm and cottonseed oil.

- **Peanuts and peanut butter** that contain hydrogenated, hardened oils and any peanuts with mold and all molds that can cause allergies.

- **Margarine** – combines heart-deadly trans-fatty acids and saturated fats.

- **Saturated fats and hydrogenated oils** – enemies that clog the arteries.

- **Coffee, soft drinks, teas, alcohol, sugared juices** – even if decaffeinated.

- **Fresh pork / products.** • **Fried, fatty, greasy meats.** • **Irradiated GMO foods.**

- **Smoked meats**, such as ham, bacon, sausage and all smoked fish.

- **Luncheon meats**, hot dogs, salami, bologna, corned beef, pastrami and packaged meats containing dangerous sodium nitrate or nitrite.

- **Dried fruits** containing sulphur dioxide – a toxic preservative.

- **Chickens, turkeys and meats injected with hormones** or fed with commercial feed containing any drugs or toxins.

- **Canned soups** – read labels for sugar, salt, starch, flour and preservatives.

- **Foods containing preservatives, additives,** benzoate of soda, salt, sugar, cream of tartar, drugs, irradiated and genetically engineered foods.

- **Day-old cooked vegetables**, potatoes and pre-mixed, wilted lifeless salads.

- **All commercial vinegars:** pasteurized, filtered, distilled, white, malt and synthetic vinegars are dead vinegars! (We use only unfiltered, organic Apple Cider Vinegar with "Mother Enzyme" as used in olden times.)

Please follow The Bragg Healthy Lifestyle to provide the basic, healthy nourishment to maintain your precious health.

The Miracle Powers of Fresh Organic Fruits

Always keep in mind that the most perfect food for man is fresh, ripe organic fruit. Mother Nature, in her unique way, brings together in fruits a marvelous balance. The fruits are living combinations of vital principles, in high rates of vibration, bio-magnetized, to release the living building blocks so necessary to maintain your life!

Tinted by basking in the rays of the vitalizing sun, taking in drafts of magnetized air, drawing into itself vital minerals through its roots in the earth, delicious, organic fruits are God's perfect creations for man!

Man can duplicate the natural occurring chemicals of an apple in a chemist's dish, but he can't construct an apple! Man may analyze the minerals of a cherry, but he doesn't know what makes it red. He may take apart and try to reconstruct a grape, and find that the grape supports life, but the man-made chemicals do not!

Fruits contain bioelectric principles that give the electric sparks of life! **Organic fruits are the most perfect foods from Mother Nature and God.** Fruits will support life indefinitely to a superior degree when a body is cleansed and living in a healthy environment. Seek out healthy organically grown produce!

Who has not had his mouth water when seeing a luscious dish of delicious, ripe fruit before him – for instance some yellow pears with a dash of pink or a beautiful bunch of tapering grapes, green, blue or red. The sight of fruits and the taste of them, more so, bring an abundant secretion of digestive juices, for fruits are the most natural foods! We can say without reserve that fruits are designed beautifully for our digestive tracts!

We have seen a sick person turn down all other foods for some freshly squeezed orange juice. His sick body craved the nutrients in juicy oranges. We have seen children torn with fever ask for fruit juice. Why didn't they ask for a hot dog? Our Mother Nature's guidance was in full force!

Junk foods, processed meats, sugar and fast foods can increase inflammation in your body which could lead to chronic diseases.
– Dr. Bob Martin, radio host and author of "Secret Nerve Cures"
www.DoctorBob.com • Patricia was a frequent guest on his radio show

But diets that consist solely of fruits are impractical for the average American, although they would be splendid for short periods in a tropical climate. While we have come so far from our natural state that we can't maintain an efficient lifestyle as 100% fruitarians, we still need to eat plenty of fresh fruits! One of the many reasons we love Hawaii are the luscious tropical fruits!

We especially recommend ripe organic bananas, which are not a fattening fruit – as many thought. They are 70% water and are high in potassium. Organic apples of all kinds make excellent eating, as do pears, oranges and grapes. In the fall, winter and spring, eat organically grown dates, sun-dried figs, raisins, apricots, etc. along with fresh fruits. When you eat fruits, see how light and wonderful you feel and look and your energy zooms!

Eat More Healthy Fiber for Super Health

❥ EAT ALL VARIETIES OF BERRIES, surprisingly good sources of fiber.

❥ KEEP BEANS HANDY, probably the best fiber sources. Cook dried beans and freeze in portions. Use canned beans for faster meals.

❥ INSTEAD OF ICEBERG LETTUCE, choose deep green lettuces (romaine, bib, butter, etc.), spinach or cabbage for variety salads.

❥ "100% NON-GMO WHOLE WHEAT" or whole grain breads. A dark color isn't proof; check labels, compare fibers, grains, etc.

❥ NON-GMO WHOLE GRAIN CEREALS. Hot, also cold granolas.

❥ GO FOR THE BROWN RICES. It's better for you and so delicious.

❥ EAT THE SKINS of potatoes and other fruits and vegetables.

❥ LOOK FOR CRACKERS with at least 2 grams of fiber per ounce.

❥ SERVE HUMMUS, made from chickpeas, instead of sour-cream dips.

❥ USE NON-GMO WHOLE WHEAT FLOUR for baking breads, muffins, pancakes, waffles and for variety try other whole grain flours.

❥ DON'T UNDERESTIMATE CORN, especially popcorn & corn tortillas.

❥ ADD NON-GMO OAT BRAN, WHEAT BRAN AND WHEATGERM to baked goods, cookies, etc.; whole grain cereals, casseroles, loafs, etc.

❥ SNACK ON SUN-DRIED FRUIT, such as apricots, dates, prunes, raisins, etc., which are concentrated sources of nutrients and fiber.

❥ INSTEAD OF DRINKING JUICE, blend fruit: orange, grapefruit, etc.; and vegetables: tomato, carrot, etc. – www.BerkeleyWellness.com

Plant-Based Protein Chart

BEANS & LEGUMES

(1 cup cooked)	PROTEIN IN GRAMS
Soybeans	29
Lentils	18
Adzuki Beans	17
Cannellini	17
Navy Beans	16
Split Peas	16
Black Beans	15
Garbanzos (chick peas)	15
Kidney Beans	15
Great Northern Beans	15
Lima Beans	15
Black-eyed Peas	14
Pinto Beans	14
Mung Beans	14
Tofu (3 oz.)	7 to 12
Green Peas (whole)	9

RAW NUTS & SEEDS

(1/4 cup or 4 Tbsps.)	PROTEIN IN GRAMS
Chia Seeds	12
Macadamia Nuts	11
Flax Seeds	8
Sunflower Seeds	8
Almonds	7
Pumpkin Seeds	7
Sesame Seeds	7
Walnuts	5
Brazil Nuts	5
Hazelnuts	5
Pine Nuts	4
Cashews	4

NUT BUTTERS

(2 Tbsps.)	PROTEIN IN GRAMS
Peanut Butter	7 to 9
Almond Butter	5 to 8
Cashew Butter	4 to 5
Sesame - Tahini	6

VEGETABLES

(1 Serving or 1 cup)	PROTEIN IN GRAMS
Spirulina	8.6
Corn (1 cob)	5
Potato (with skin)	5
Mushrooms, Oyster	5
Artichoke (1 medium)	4
Collard Greens	4
Broccoli	4
Brussel Sprouts	4
Mushrooms, Shiitake	3.5
Swiss Chard	3
Kale	2.5
Asparagus (5 spears)	2
String Beans	2
Beets	2
Peas	2
Sweet Potato	3
Summer Squash	2
Cabbage	2
Carrot	2
Cauliflower	2
Squash	2
Celery	1
Spinach	1
Bell Peppers	1
Cucumber	1
Eggplant	1
Leeks	1
Lettuce	1
Tomato (1 medium)	1
Radish	1
Turnips	1

DAIRY & NUT MILKS

(1 cup)	PROTEIN IN GRAMS
Oat Milk	3 to 4
Almond Milk	1 to 2
Rice Milk	1
Eggs (1) *(free-range)*	6

FRUITS

(1 Serving or 1 cup)	PROTEIN IN GRAMS
Avocado (1 medium)	4
Banana (1)	1 to 2
Blackberries (1 cup)	2
Pomegranate (1)	1.5
Blueberries (1 cup)	1
Cantaloupe (1 cup)	1
Cherries (1 cup)	1
Grapes (1 cup)	1
Honeydew (1 cup)	1
Kiwi (1 large)	1
Lemon (1)	1
Mango (1)	1
Nectarine (1)	1
Orange (1)	1
Peach (1)	1
Pear (1)	1
Pineapple (1 cup)	1
Plum (1)	1
Raspberries (1 cup)	1
Strawberries (1 cup)	1
Watermelon (1 cup)	1

GRAINS & RICE

(1 cup cooked)	PROTEIN IN GRAMS
Triticale	25
Millet	8.4
Amaranth	7
Oat Bran	7
Wild Rice	7
Couscous (whole wheat)	6
Bulgur Wheat	6
Buckwheat	6
Teff	6
Oat Groats	6
Barley	5
Quinoa	5
Brown Rice	5
Spelt	5

69

This chart displays protein content of common vegetarian foods.
Note that in order to determine amount of protein that is optimal for your body, use the following formula that is based on a vegan diet: *RDA recommends that we take in 0.36 grams of protein per pound that we weigh* (100 lbs. x 0.36 = 36 grams).

Data from webs: *TheHolyKale.com • VegParadise.com • vrg.org (Vegetarian Resource Group).*

Food and Product Summary

Today, many of our foods are highly processed or refined, robbing them of essential nutrients, vitamins, minerals and enzymes! Many also contain harmful, toxic and dangerous chemicals! The research findings and experience of top nutritionists, physicians and dentists have led to the discovery that devitalized foods are a major cause of poor health, illness, cancer and premature death. The enormous increase in the last 70 years of degenerative diseases such as heart disease, arthritis, diabetes and dental decay, verify this belief. Scientific research has shown that most of these afflictions can be prevented and that others, once established, can be arrested or even reversed through nutritional and healthy lifestyle methods.

Enjoy Super Health with Natural Foods

1. **RAW FOODS:** Fresh fruits and raw vegetables organically grown are always best! Enjoy nutritious variety garden salads with raw vegetables, sprouts, raw nuts and seeds.

2. **VEGETABLES and PROTEINS:**
   a. Legumes, lentils, brown rice, and all beans.
   b. Nuts and seeds, raw and unsalted (lightly roasted is okay).
   c. We prefer healthier vegetarian proteins. If you eat animal protein, then be sure it's hormone-free, and organically fed and no more than 1 or 2 times a week.
   d. Dairy products – fertile range-free eggs, unprocessed hard cheese and feta goat's cheese. We choose not to use dairy products. Try healthier non-dairy rice, coconut, and almond milks and non-dairy cheeses and delicious rice and oat ice cream.

3. **FRUITS and VEGETABLES:** Organically grown is always best, grown without the use of poisonous sprays and toxic chemical fertilizers. Urge markets to stock organic produce! Steam, bake, sauté and wok vegetables as short a time as possible to retain the best nutritional content and flavor. Also enjoy fresh juices.

4. **ORGANIC non-GMO WHOLE GRAINS, CEREALS, BREADS:** They contain important B-Complex vitamins, vitamin E, minerals, fiber and the important unsaturated fatty acids.

5. **COLD or EXPELLER-PRESSED VEGETABLE OILS:** Organic, first press, extra virgin olive oil (is best), coconut, avocado, flax, and sesame oils are good sources of healthy, essential, unsaturated fatty acids. We still use oils sparingly.

Mother Nature's Miracle Phytochemicals Help Prevent Cancer

Make sure to get your daily dose of naturally occurring, cancer-fighting super foods – phytochemicals are abundant in apples, tomatoes, onions, garlic, beans, legumes, soybeans, cabbage, cauliflower, broccoli, citrus, etc. Champions with highest count of phytochemicals – apples and tomatoes.

Phytochemical	Food Sources	Health Action
PHYTOESTROGEN ISOFLAVONES	Soy products, flaxseed, seeds and nuts, yams, alfalfa, pomegranates lentils, carrots, apples	Helps block some cancers, aids in menopausal symptoms, balances hormones, helps improve memory, enhances heart health
PHYTOSTEROLS	Plant oils: corn, sesame, safflower; rice bran, wheat germ, peanuts	Blocks hormonal role in cancers, inhibits uptake of cholesterol from diet, reduce risk of heart attack
LIGNANS	Flaxseeds, rye, lentils, soy mushrooms, barley	Helps prevent breast cancer, heart disease and balances hormones
SAPONINS	Yams, beets, beans, cabbage, nuts, soybeans	Helps prevent cancer cells from multiplying, reduces cholesterol
TERPENES	Carrots, winter squash, sweet potatoes, yams, apples, cantaloupes, cherries	Antioxidants – protects DNA from free radical-induced damage, and improves immunity
	Tomatoes and its sauces, tomato-based products	Helps block UVA & UVB and offers help to protect against cancers – breast, prostate, etc.
	Spinach, kale, beet and turnip greens, cabbage	Protects eyes from macular degeneration,
	Red chile peppers	Keeps carcinogens from binding to DNA
QUERCETIN (& FLAVONOIDS)	Apples (especially the skins), red onions and green tea	Strong cancer fighter, protects heart - arteries. Reduces pain, allergy and asthma symptoms
	Citrus fruits (flavonoids)	Promotes protective enzymes
PHENOLS	Apples, fennel, parsley, carrots, alfalfa, cabbage	Helps prevent blood clotting & has important anticancer properties
	Cinnamon	Promotes healthy blood sugar and glucose metabolism
	Citrus fruits, broccoli, cabbage, cucumbers, green peppers, tomatoes	Antioxidants – flavonoids, block membrane receptor sites for certain hormones
	Apples, grape seeds	Strong antioxidants; fights germs and bacteria, strengthens immune system, veins and capillaries
	Grapes, especially skins	Antioxidant, antimutagen; promotes detoxification. Acts as carcinogen inhibitors
	Yellow and green squash	Antihepatotoxic, antitumor
SULFUR COMPOUNDS	Onions and garlic, (fresh is always best) Red onions (our favorite) also contain Quercetin Onions help keep doctor away	Promotes liver enzymes, inhibits cholesterol synthesis, reduces triglycerides, lowers blood pressure improves immune response, fights infections, germs and parasites

71

HEALTHY BEVERAGES
Fresh Juices, Herb Teas & Energy Drinks

These freshly squeezed organic vegetable and fruit juices are important to *The Bragg Healthy Lifestyle*. It's not wise to drink beverages with your main meals, as it dilutes the digestive juices. But it's great during the day to have a glass of freshly squeezed orange juice, grapefruit juice, vegetable juice, raw, organic apple cider vinegar drink (see below), or herbal tea – these are all ideal pick-me-up beverages.

Apple Cider Vinegar Drink – Mix 1-2 tsps. raw, unfiltered organic apple cider vinegar (with the 'Mother' enzyme) and (optional) to taste raw honey or pure maple syrup *(if diabetic, to sweeten use 2 stevia drops)* in 8 oz. of distilled or purified water. Take glass upon arising, an hour before lunch and dinner.

Delicious Hot or Cold Cider Drink – Add 2-3 cinnamon sticks and 4 cloves to water and boil. Steep 20 minutes or more. Before serving add raw, unfiltered organic apple cider vinegar and sweetener to taste.

Favorite Juice Drink – This drink consists of all raw organic vegetables which we prepare in our juicer / blender: carrots, celery, cucumber, beets, cabbage, tomatoes, watercress, kale, parsley, or any vegetable combination you prefer. The great purifier, garlic we enjoy, but it's optional.

Bragg's Favorite Healthy Energy Smoothie – After our morning stretch and exercises we often enjoyed the drink below instead of fruit. It's a delicious and powerfully nutritious meal anytime: lunch, dinner, or take in a thermos to work, school, sports, gym, hiking, or the park. You can freeze for it for popsicles too.

72

Bragg's Favorite Healthy Energy Smoothie

Prepare the following in a blender, add frozen juice cubes if desired colder; Choice of: freshly squeezed orange or grapefruit juice; carrot and greens juice; unsweetened pineapple juice; or $1^1/2$ - 2 cups purified or distilled water with:

2 tsps. spirulina or green powder	*1-2 bananas or fresh fruit*
$1/3$ tsp. Nutritional Yeast	*1-2 tsps. almond or nut butter*
2 dates or prunes-pitted	*1 tsp. flaxseed oil or ground seeds*
1 tsp. protein powder (optional)	*1 tsp. raw honey (optional)*

Optional: 4-6 apricots (sun-dried,) soak in jar overnight in purified water or unsweetened pineapple juice. We soak enough to last for several days. Keep refrigerated. In summer you can add organic fresh fruit: peaches, papaya, blueberries, strawberries, all berries, apricots, etc. instead of banana. In winter, add apples, kiwi, oranges, tangelos, persimmons or pears, and if fresh is unavailable, try sugar-free, frozen organic fruits. Serves 1 to 2.

Patricia's Delicious Health Popcorn

Use freshly popped organic popcorn (use air popper). Drizzle organic olive oil, melted coconut oil or salt-free butter over popcorn. Sprinkle with good quality nutritional yeast for amazing flavor. For a variety try a pinch of cayenne pepper, mustard powder or fresh crushed garlic to oil mixture. Serve instead of breads!

Healthy, healing dietary fibers are organic fresh vegetables, fruits, salads whole grains and their products. These health builders help normalize your blood pressure, cholesterol and promotes healthy elimination.

Lentil & Brown Rice Casserole, Burgers or Soup
Paul Bragg and Jack LaLanne's Favorite Recipe

16 oz pkg organic lentils, uncooked
1 cup brown organic rice, uncooked
5 cups, distilled / purified water
4-6 carrots, chop $^1/_2$" rounds
3 celery stalks, chop

4 garlic cloves, chop
2 onions, chop
2 tsps. organic coconut aminos
1 tsp. salt-free all-purpose seasoning
2 tsps. organic extra-virgin olive oil

1 cup diced fresh or canned tomatoes (salt-free)

Wash and drain lentils and rice. Place grains in large stainless steel pot. Add water, bring to boil, reduce heat and simmer 30 minutes. Now add vegetables and seasonings and cook on low heat until tender. Last five minutes add fresh or canned (salt-free) tomatoes. For delicious garnish, add minced parsley. **For Burgers mash. For Soup, add more water in cooking grains.** Serves 4 to 6.

Raw Organic Vegetable Health Salad

2 stalks celery, chop
1 bell pepper & seeds, dice
$^1/_2$ cucumber, slice
2 carrots, grate
1 raw beet, grate
1 cup green cabbage, chop

$^1/_2$ cup red cabbage, chop
$^1/_2$ cup alfalfa, mung or sunflower sprouts
2 spring onions & green tops, chop
1 turnip, grate
1 avocado (ripe)
3 tomatoes, medium size

For variety add organic raw zucchini, peas, mushrooms, broccoli, cauliflower, (try black olives and pasta). Chop, slice or grate vegetables fine to medium for variety in size. Mix vegetables & serve on bed of lettuce, spinach, chopped kale or cabbage. Dice avocado and tomato and serve on side as a dressing. Serve choice of fresh squeezed lemon, orange or dressing separately. Chill salad plates before serving. **It's best to always eat salad first before hot dishes.** Serves 3 to 5.

73

Patricia's Health Salad Dressing

$^1/_2$ cup raw organic apple cider vinegar
1-2 tsps. organic raw honey
$^1/_3$ cup organic extra-virgin olive oil, or blend with safflower, sesame or flax oil
1 Tbsp. fresh herbs, minced (to taste)

$^1/_2$ tsp. organic coconut aminos
1-2 cloves garlic, minced

Blend ingredients in blender or jar. Refrigerate in covered jar.

For delicious Herbal Vinegar: In a quart jar add $^1/_3$ cup tightly packed, crushed fresh sweet basil, tarragon, dill, oregano, or any fresh herbs desired, combined or singly (If dried herbs, use 1-2 tsps. herbs). Now cover to top with raw, organic apple cider vinegar and store two weeks in warm place, and then strain and refrigerate.

Honey – Chia or Celery Seed Vinaigrette

$^1/_4$ tsp. dry mustard
$^1/_4$ tsp. organic coconut aminos
$^1/_4$ tsp. paprika or to taste
1-2 Tbsps. honey

1 cup organic apple cider vinegar
$^1/_2$ cup organic extra-virgin olive oil
$^1/_2$ small onion, minced
$^1/_3$ tsp. chia or celery seed (or vary to taste)

Blend ingredients in blender or jar. Refrigerate in covered jar.

Studies show both beta carotene and vitamin C, abundantly found in fruits and vegetables, play vital roles in preventing heart disease and cancers.

Allergies & Dr. Coca's Pulse Test

Almost every known food may cause some allergic reaction at times. Thus, foods used in *elimination* diets may cause allergic reactions in some individuals. Some are listed among the *Most Common Food Allergies* (see next page). Since reaction to these foods is generally low, they are widely used in making test diets. By keeping a food journal and tracking your pulse rate after meals you will soon know your *problem* foods. Allergic foods cause pulse to then go up. (Take base pulse, for 1 minute, before meals, then 30 minutes after meals, and also before bed. If it increases 8-10 beats per minute – check foods for allergies.)

If your body has a reaction after eating some particular food, especially if it happens each time you eat that food, you may have an allergy. Some allergic reactions are: wheezing, sneezing, stuffy nose, nasal drip or mucus, dark circles, eye watering or bags under your eyes, headaches, feeling light-headed or dizzy, fast heart beat, stomach or chest pains, diarrhea, extreme thirst, breaking out in a rash, swelling of extremities or stomach bloating. **Do read Dr. Arthur Coca's book, *The Pulse Test.***

74

If you know what you're allergic to, you are lucky; if you don't, you had better find out as fast as possible and eliminate all irritating foods from your diet. To re-evaluate your daily life and have a health guide to your future, start a daily journal (keep a notebook – enlarge and copy form on page 76) of foods eaten, your pulse rate before and after meals and your reactions, moods, energy levels, weight, elimination and sleep patterns. You will discover the foods and situations causing problems. **By charting your diet you will be amazed at the effects of eating certain foods. We have kept daily journals for years.**

If you are hypersensitive to certain foods, you must omit them from your diet! There are hundreds of allergies and of course it's impossible here to take up each one. Many have allergies to milk, wheat, or some are allergic to all grains. **Visit web: *FoodAllergy.org*. Your daily journal will help you discover and accurately pinpoint the foods and situations causing you problems. Start your journal today!**

Most Common Food Allergies

- **DAIRY:** Butter, Cheese, Cottage Cheese, Ice Cream, Milk, Yogurt, etc.
- **CEREALS & GRAINS:** Wheat, Corn, Buckwheat, Oats, Rye
- **EGGS:** Cakes, Custards, Dressings, Mayonnaise, Noodles
- **FISH:** Shellfish, Crabs, Lobster, Shrimp, Shad Roe
- **MEATS:** Bacon, Beef, Chicken, Pork, Sausage, Veal, Smoked Products
- **FRUITS:** Citrus Fruits, Melons, Strawberries
- **NUTS:** Peanuts, Pecans, Walnuts, chemically dried preserved nuts
- **MISCELLANEOUS:** Chocolate, Cocoa, Coffee, Black & Green (caffeine) Teas, Palm & Cottonseed Oils, MSG & Salt.

"Gardenburger" Creator Thanks Bragg Books

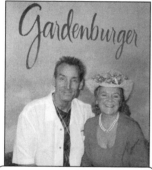

Patricia with Paul Wenner

Paul Wenner, the Gardenburger Creator, says his early years as a youth with asthma were so bad he would stand at the window praying to breathe through the night and stay alive. A miracle happened when as a teenager he read the Bragg Books *The Miracle of Fasting* and *Bragg Healthy Lifestyle* and his years of asthma were cured in only one month. Paul became so inspired that he wanted to be a Health Crusader like Paul Bragg and his daughter Patricia – and Paul Wenner did! Gardenburgers are sold worldwide and were one of the first meatless burgers! *GardenBurger.com*

75

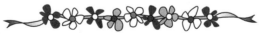

An allergy no longer means merely hay-fever, asthma or an outbreak of hives. It can also mean high blood pressure, diabetes, epileptic seizures and stammering. It means "that tired feeling," constipation, stomach ulcer, dizzy spells, headaches and mental depression. In truth, it may mean much of what ails the health and happiness of human beings.
  – Arthur F. Coca, M.D., author, "The Pulse Test" • SoilAndHealth.org

---

I now live on legumes, vegetables and fruits. No dairy, no meat of any kind, no chicken, no turkey, and very little fish, only once in a while. It changed my metabolism and I lost 24 pounds. I did research and found 82% of people who go on plant-based diet begin to heal themselves, as I did.
  – Bill Clinton, United States President, 1993-2001

MY DAILY HEALTH JOURNAL

Today is:____/____/____

> *I have said my morning resolve and am ready to practice faithfully The Bragg Healthy Lifestyle today and every day.*

Yesterday I went to bed at: Today I arose at: Weight:

Today I practiced the No-Heavy Breakfast or No-Breakfast Plan: ☐ yes ☐ no

• For Breakfast I drank: Time:

  For Breakfast I ate:

                                                               Time:

  Supplements:

• For Lunch I ate: Time:

  Supplements:

• For Dinner I ate: Time:

  Supplements:

• ____ Glasses of Water I Drank during the Day, including ACV Drinks

  List Snacks – Type and When:

_____

• I took part in these physical activities (walking, gym, etc.) today:

_____

Grade each on scale of 1 to 10 (desired optimum health is 10).

• I rate my day for the following categories:

Previous Night's Sleep:	Stress/Anxiety:
Energy Level:	Elimination:
Physical Activity, Exercise:	Health:
Peacefulness:	Accomplishments:
Happiness:	Self-Esteem:

_____

• General Comments, Reactions and any To-Do List:

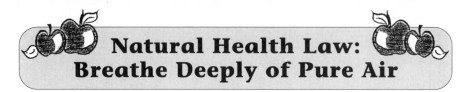

Natural Health Law:
Breathe Deeply of Pure Air

Oxygen is The Invisible Staff of Life

Oxygen is the life of the blood, and blood is the life of the body! Oxygen is the most important element in the body! It is colorless, odorless and tasteless. Its main function is purification. Lack of oxygen in the body can lead to serious consequences. The majority of people are oxygen starved because they are shallow breathers. See *Bragg Super Power Breathing* book.

To have a healthy, youthful, vital life, we need fresh, unpolluted air in abundance, purified distilled water and fresh organic vegetables and fruits. Remember, ample oxygen is an unquestionable source of indispensable energy necessary for higher vital activity in the human organism! It helps you ensure healthier elimination, reconstruction and regeneration within the vital factors and metabolic activities of the entire physical body!

Through the lung functioning, oxygen is absorbed and assimilated into the bloodstream, bringing with it other unknown factors from the atmosphere. Plants, through their roots, absorb the vital elements in the soil necessary for their life. If we cut or damage their roots, they die! **Man's roots are his lungs!** Smokers are killing their lungs and the lungs of all those around them! Don't be around secondhand smoke – it's even more deadly! Allow no smoking in your home! See dangers of smoking in *Bragg Super Power Breathing* Book.

The oxygen in the air that we breathe helps dissolve and eliminate the waste and builds the continuum of our cellular structure! This maintains our body to the highest degree possible! Each breath should detoxify and regenerate our vital forces. But this rejuvenation process must be supplemented by faithfully following The Bragg Healthy Lifestyle. Please understand that both exercise and deep breathing must be fortified with proper healthy nutritious food to prevent degenerative and destructive premature breakdown of your 38 trillion cells.

Here's Health Benefits of Deep Breathing
and Why You Should Make it a Part of Your Daily Living!

♣ **Deep Breathing Detoxifies and Releases Toxins.** The body is designed to release 70% of its toxins through breathing. If you are not breathing in pure air effectively, you are not ridding your body of toxins. The more toxic poison you burn, the more vitality you will create!

♣ **All Internal Organs are Massaged.** Movements of the diaphragm during deep breathing exercise massage the stomach, small intestine, liver and the pancreas.

♣ **Respiratory System Works Better.** Respiratory diseases like asthma, bronchitis, Chronic Obstructive Pulmonary Disease, emphysema and even chest pain can subside.

♣ **Digestive System Does Its Job.** Digestive ills (poor digestion, bloating, constipation) are helped by the internal massage of correct diaphragmatic action. When Super Power Breath is taken, your digestive tract gets healthy exercise. **Deep optimal breathing is the great body health normalizer. Oxygen, the invisible staff of life, is food for the body and helps with assimilation of foods. Oxygen burns calories and helps promote normal, healthy weight.** The digestive organs receive more oxygen, and hence operate more efficiently.

♣ **Lymph System Works Better.** Increases circulation of lymphatic fluid which speeds recovery after illnesses.

♣ **Circulation System Moves!** Many people suffer from poor circulation in various parts of the body. Because they don't get sufficient oxygen to produce a steady blood circulation into their extremities, they have cold hands, feet, noses and ears. **The more oxygen you get into your body, the better it is for your circulation, heart, and your hands and feet will be warmer!** When more oxygen gets into your bloodstream, you will feel super energized and have greater super vitality to better enjoy a longer, healthier, happier life! *Breathing.com*

Breathing is the greatest pleasure in life – it gives life!
– Giovanni Papini, Italian journalist, poet and novelist 1881-1956

Breathing is our connection to life, through the body and heart, leading us to a wholeness of being and giving us spirit for living life to its fullest.

❀ **Immune System has More Energy. Deep Breathing creates more energy for the body to heal and detoxify.** Helps tissues to regenerate and heal. Enriches your blood cells to metabolize nutrients and vitamins. Super Power Breathing is now a part of all cures. In the modern hospital, pure oxygen heals when every other method of healing has failed. Even broken bones heal more quickly when blood is purified by doing daily Super Power Breathing Exercises. Oxygen – the great invisible food for life, stimulant and purifier – builds our health resistance to infections and strengthens our weak points. It's our most vital aid in helping the body to heal itself and to stay healthy!

❀ **Cleansing Systems Works Better.** Excess fluids are eliminated through deep breathing. The stress on organs is lessened, allowing the body to cleanse naturally.

❀ **Blood Quality Improves.** When you regularly breathe oxygen correctly, you add millions of health-giving, oxygen-carrying red blood cells to your bloodstream, your miracle river of life. Deep Breathing removes all the carbon-dioxide and increases oxygen in the blood.

79

❀ **Nervous System Improves.** Brain, spinal cord and nerves receive increased oxygen. This improves the health of the whole body, since the nervous system communicates to all parts of the body. Many nervous diseases are due to oxygen starvation. Deep, diaphragmatic breathing tranquilizes jangled nerves, stimulates the brain with clear thinking and more alertness to help solve any life problems and to help you make wise decisions.

❀ **Lungs are Strengthened.** When you fill your lungs with more miracle-working oxygen, you cleanse your body of toxic poisons that could do your body great health damage. As you breathe deeply lungs become healthier and more powerful. Good insurance against respiratory problems.

Other factors affecting breathing: Our thoughts and emotions interfere with our breathing. That's why, with a headache or some other sudden symptom, a few minutes of slow, deep breathing exercises will help you detoxify and reestablish healthy internal balance and blood pressure.

✿ **Heart Grows Stronger.** Slow, deep breaths soothe and recharge the heart. Conversely, rapid, shallow breathing exhausts it through overwork and lack of sufficient oxygen for the blood. Since the heart doesn't have to work as hard to deliver oxygen to tissues, the heart can rest a little.

✿ **Muscles Get a Workout.** When you breathe easier you move easier! Deep breathing increases flexibility and strengthens joints. Supplies oxygen to brain and all cells in your body which increases the muscles in your body.

✿ **Emotionally You Feel Better.** People who deeply inhale larger amounts of oxygen are happier people. Super Power Breathing cleanses your body of psychological and physical poisons and gives you more joyful daily living and also more emotional well-being.

✿ **Reduces Feelings of Stress.** Deep breathing relaxes the body and releases endorphins – natural pain-killers that create natural highs – and makes it easier to sleep. Deep breathing helps clear uneasy feelings out of your body.

✿ **Become Mentally Present.** Mental observation and concentration improves. There is greater productivity, insight and learning and better decision making.

✿ **Physical Appearance Improves.** People who get ample oxygen sleep better and have better muscle tone. Skin is healthier, firmer and more alive! Oxygen is Mother Nature's great miracle beautifier. It gives the skin a radiant glow and the hair a lustrous sheen. You will have fewer wrinkles from improved circulation. Breathing helps create beautiful skin at any age! Good breathing techniques will also encourage good posture, which in turn helps you to look and feel younger (see posture exercise page 88). If you are overweight, the extra oxygen helps burn up excess fat more efficiently.

✿ **Increases Spirituality.** Deep Breathing deepens your meditation and increases intuition when you're relaxed. Helps connect you to your inner soul which helps with "self-love" and greater compassion for others.

✿ **Promotes Super Energy!** You will no longer crave artificial stimulants (caffeine, alcohol, tobacco) when sufficient oxygen is taken into your system. Oxygen is the wise stimulant that has no harmful after-effects.

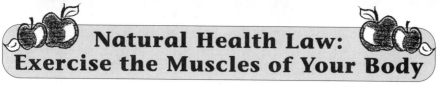

Natural Health Law:
Exercise the Muscles of Your Body

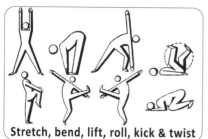

Stretch, bend, lift, roll, kick & twist

To ensure youthful arteries, exercise is very essential! If you wish to live and enjoy a long, fit and healthy life it's necessary to build up your cardiovascular endurance and start now to follow an exercise program designed to keep your arteries unclogged, soft, agile and healthy. The first step is to get more oxygen into the body which will help dissolve the encrustations that have formed in the arteries. Any physical activity that injects more oxygen is going to help extend your life!

Enjoy a Tireless – Ageless – Pain-free Body as Conrad Hilton, J.C. Penney & Dr. Scholl Did With The Bragg Healthy Lifestyle

81

Don't despair in your golden years – enjoy them! My dad Paul C. Bragg, said *life's second half is the best* and can be the most healthy fruitful years. Linus Pauling, painter Grandma Moses and amazing Mother Teresa, have all proven that! These three famous Bragg Health Followers – Conrad Hilton, J.C. Penney and foot Doctor Scholl were all Bragg health followers and lived strong, productive, active lives into their 90's. Countless others have lived long, healthy fulfilled lives following The Bragg Healthy Lifestyle, you can too!

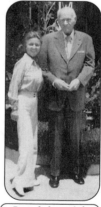

Patricia with Conrad Hilton

We teach you how to forget calendar years and to regain not only a youthful spirit, but much of the vigor of your youth. It's your duty to yourself to start to live a healthy life today – don't procrastinate! Keep premature ageing out of your body by faithfully living this healthy lifestyle blueprint. You must eat foods that have a high health vibration rate (abundance of raw, organic fruits and vegetables) and do a water fast weekly.

Also, do Bragg Super Power Deep Breathing exercises, and get eight hours of optimal sleep at night. Don't let anything rob you of your emotional and nervous energy and precious vital force! Do read *Bragg Building Powerful Nerve Force & Positive Energy* and *Super Power Breathing* Books.

Your body is being made anew every day! Premature ageing and senility result from the toxic debris that accumulates when you live an unhealthy lifestyle. Now eat right, exercise for good body circulation, and there will be little or no buildup of toxins to clog and prematurely age your body. Cultivate and hold onto the spirit of youth *and it will be yours!* You can feel and look younger! Practice good posture to maintain health and energy. Daily do The Bragg Posture Exercise on page 88. Follow The Bragg Healthy Lifestyle and you will be blessed with many miracles!

If you're already in the clutches of premature ageing, begin now to fight for the return of youthfulness! Work to restore your priceless possession! You can do it! Train your body as you would that of a race horse. Follow these clear, definite instructions and you will gain strength, virility, energy, vivacity and enthusiasm! Make your life a daily enjoyment of the most precious of all earthly gifts – the power and joys of youthful, healthful living. Men and women can be young at 60, 70, 80 and even 90. Some have retained the spirit of youth beyond the century mark.

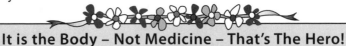

It is the Body – Not Medicine – That's The Hero!

"It is the body that is the hero, not science, not antibiotics . . . not machines, drugs or new devices. The task of the physician today is what it has always been, to help the body do what it has learned so well to do on its own during its unending struggle for survival to heal itself!"
– Ronald Glasser, M.D., author of "The Body is The Hero"

It's never too late to get into shape, but it does take daily perseverance.
– Dr. Thomas K. Cureton – Physical Fitness Pioneer, University of Illinois

Each patient carries his own doctor inside him. – Albert Schweitzer, M.D.

Making positive lifestyle changes – healthy eating, deep breathing, daily exercise, fasting and eliminating stress – lowers heart disease risk.
– Johns Hopkins Medical News • www.HopkinsMedicine.org

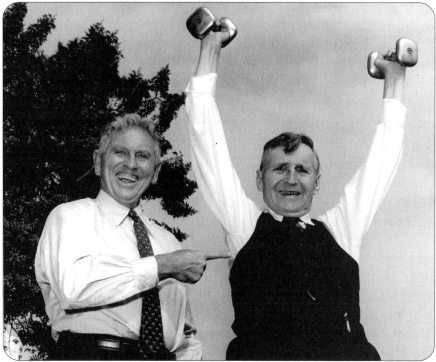

Paul Bragg and Weight-lifting Health Follower, Roy White

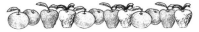
83

Exercise and ACV Helps Keep You More Youthful, Healthier, Stronger, Flexible and Trim

Paul and Roy practiced progressive weight training three times a week to stay healthy and fit. Scientists have proven that weight training works miracles for all ages by maintaining more flexibility, energy and youthful stamina!

Iron Pumping Oldsters (86 to 96) Triple Their Muscle Strength in U.S. Study

WASHINGTON – Ageing nursing home residents in Boston study "pumping iron?" Elderly weight-lifters tripling and quadrupling their muscle strength? Is it possible? Most people would doubt it! But government experts on ageing answered those questions with a resounding "yes" thanks to the results of this amazing landmark study!

Age does not depend upon years, but upon lifestyle and health!

You are what you Eat, Drink, Breathe, Think, Say & Do. – Patricia Bragg

They turned a group of frail Boston nursing home residents, aged 86 to 96, into weight-lifters to demonstrate that it's never too late to reverse age-related decline in muscle strength. The group participated in a regimen of high-intensity weight-training in a study conducted by Dr. Maria A. Fiatarone at Tufts University in Boston.

Amazing Strength Results in 8 Weeks

"The favorable response to strength training in our subjects was remarkable in light of their advanced ages and sedentary habits. The elderly weight-lifters increased their muscle strength by three-fold to four-fold in as little as eight weeks." Dr. Fiatarone said they were stronger at the end of the program than they had been in years! The results were amazing! Dr. Fiatarone and associates emphasized the safety of such a closely supervised weight-lifting program, even among people in frail health. The average age of the participants was 90. Six had coronary heart disease; seven had arthritis; six had bone fractures resulting from osteoporosis; four had high blood pressure; and all had been physically inactive for years. Yet, no serious medical problems resulted from the strength exercise program. A few of the participants did report minor muscle and joint aches.

The study participants, faithfully worked out 3 times a week with hand weights and weight-lifting machines. The weights were gradually increased from 10 pounds to about 40 pounds at the end of the eight week program. Dr. Fiatarone said the study carries important health implications to improve the wellness and fitness of older people, who represent a growing proportion of the U.S. population! Sadly a decline in muscle strength, tone and muscle size is the more predictable feature of ageing.

A strong body makes a strong mind. – Thomas Jefferson, 3rd U.S. President

Exercise, along with healthy foods and some fasting helps maintain or restore a healthy physical balance and normal weight for long, happy life.

❀ *Excess body fat is linked to killer diseases, such as high blood* ❀
pressure, diabetes, stroke and heart attack. Raw, apple cider vinegar contains natural occurring acetic acid, primary vinegar ingredient. Studies show it helps boost metabolism and helps to dissolve fats.

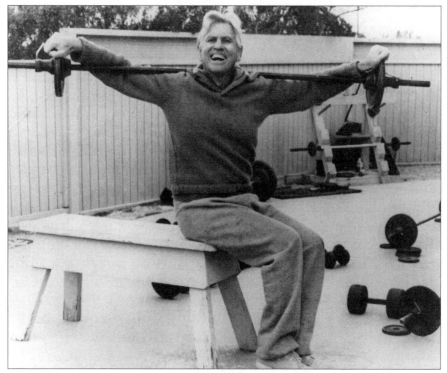

Paul and Patricia enjoyed lifting weights 3 times weekly

Building Up a Healthy Body with Exercise

Exercise helps to normalize blood pressure and create a healthy pulse. It keeps the blood flowing smoothly and not clotting. Staying active keeps you feeling energized! Brisk walking is the best all-around exercise. Vow to become a health walker daily. Along with walking, we like to encourage you to use free-weights or dumbbells to build up your muscles. Lifting weights is a great compliment to the workout your legs get from walking. Keep your weights in the living room and use them as you watch TV in the evening. Even people well into their 70's, 80's and even 90's can be weight-lifters. All you have to do is start. You'll never regret it.

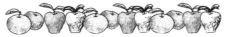

Staying active is like riding an UP elevator. The more you do, the more you feel like staying involved.

What a person eats becomes his own body chemistry.
– Paul C. Bragg, N.D., Ph.D.

Fitness Promotes Health and Longevity
It's Never Too Late to Start!

Muscle strength in the average adult decreases by 30% to 50% during the course of life, mostly consequences of a sedentary unhealthy lifestyle and other controllable factors (*diet habits, etc.*). Muscle atrophy and weakness are not merely cosmetic problems with the frail elderly. Researchers now link muscle weakness with recurrent falls, a major cause of immobility and death, sadly in the American elderly population. This is costing millions of dollars yearly in staggering medical expenses! Previous studies have also suggested weight-training can be helpful in reversing age-related muscle weakness. But Dr. Fiatarone said physicians have been reluctant to recommend weight-lifting for the frail elderly with multiple health problems. This government study might be changing their minds! This study also shows the great importance of keeping the 640 muscles as active and fit as possible to maintain general good health.

86

The Miracle Life of Jack LaLanne

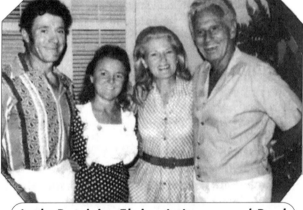

Jack, Patricia, Elaine LaLanne and Paul

Jack says he would have been dead by 17 if he hadn't attended The Bragg Crusade. Jack says, *Bragg saved my life at 15, when I attended the Bragg Health Crusade in Oakland, California.* From that day, Jack faithfully continued to live The Bragg Healthy Lifestyle, inspiring millions to health, fitness and a long and happy life! *JackLaLanne.com*

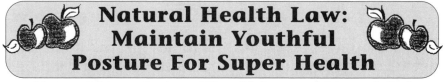

Natural Health Law: Maintain Youthful Posture For Super Health

Keep Your Spine Flexible and Youthful

One of the main keys to looking 10-20 years younger is to keep the spine active and strive for flexibility and elasticity in every part of your body, especially your spine! Also, remember to stand, walk and sit tall because all youthful-looking people have good posture!

The spine is a marvelous instrument as well as the central support of the whole body. It is made up of a flexible column of squarish bones that are joined together with rubbery puffs called discs. This wonderful piece of equipment stores its own lubrication in little sacs at the joints. The spine was designed for action! Keep it loose and supple, and your whole body will move with grace, ease and youthfulness. Read the *Bragg Back & Foot Fitness Program* book for the *Bragg Simple Spine Exercises* to help keep your spine and you flexible and youthful.

Your Waist-Line is Your Life-Line, Date-Line and Health-Line!

Get a tape measure and measure your waist. Write down the measurement. If you consciously pursue vigorous abdominal and postural exercises combined with correct eating and a weekly 24-hour fast (and later on, 3-to 7-day fasts), in a short time you'll see a more trim, youthful waist-line! Trim waist-lines make people appear years younger! Let's get yours down to where it should be, if it has grown too big. It's a trim, lean horse for the long race of life! All want longevity! Studies show ***the bigger the waist-line – the shorter the life-span!*** Living The Bragg Healthy Lifestyle is so wise and wonderful. Your life and each day is a precious gift to treasure, guard and enjoy!

People abuse their abdomens abominably! You cannot eat unhealthy, high calorie snacks and fast foods and think they won't show! Dead, devitalized foods create toxic poisons inside your body. This unhealthy over-eating all adds flabby unhealthy fat and inches to your abdomen and body.

Large Waist-Lines Lead to Shorter Life-Spans

Do not overeat even healthy foods, for your body only needs enough food (fuel) to maintain health and energy. People become overweight because they have over-fueled their bodies! Remember the studies show large waist-lines produce shorter lifespans. *www.Obesity.org*

You are not getting away with this kind of cheating, you are just hurting yourself! Bear in mind that as we live longer, the internal abdominal structure and stomach muscles relax more. This is called droopy tummy or visceroptosis. It's a common condition among older people who don't exercise their waist muscles. It can be a contributing cause of constipation, sluggish liver and even hernias. Please daily do Bragg Posture Exercise, see below.

When the abdominal wall becomes lazy and then the consequent droop is compounded by fatty layers of flab, trouble can start inside the abdomen. By the time most people reach 40, they have a prolapsed abdomen. Become a people watcher and you will notice that what we're saying is true! Some need a surgical tummy-tuck (which removes excess flab) to give them a flat stomach. So, don't let your abdominal muscles droop! Make every effort to recapture firmness. It's amazing how quickly muscles respond to exercises, sit-ups and good posture!

Bragg Posture Exercise Gives Instant Youthfulness

Stand (feet 8" apart) before a mirror and stretch up your spine. Tighten buttocks and suck in stomach muscles, lift up rib cage, put chest out, shoulders back, chin up slightly. Line body up straight (nose plumb-line straight to belly button), drop hands to sides and swing arms to normalize your posture. Do this posture exercise daily and miraculous changes will happen! You are retraining and strengthening your muscles to stand straight for health and youthfulness. Remember when you slump, you also cramp your precious machinery. This posture exercise (do 3-4 times daily) will retrain your frame to sit, stand and walk tall for health, fitness and longevity!

For those patients who have a large waist, trimming down even a few inches – through exercise and diet – could have important health benefits. – Dr. James Cerhan, Epidemiologist, Mayo Clinic • www.MayoClinic.org

Maintain Youthful Posture for Super Health

There is a fundamental relationship between good posture and youth on the one hand and between bent posture and age on the other! To maintain the posture of youth actually means to maintain youth itself, because of the basic relationship between the healthy, normal spine and bodily vigor: the condition that signifies youth, irrespective of how many years one has lived on Earth!

The most easily recognized sign of premature ageing is the forward bending of the spine, combined with "rounded shoulders" that accompany it. Prematurely old people often exhibit this condition to an extreme degree, almost bending over double. Even some school children sometimes display poor posture, stooped, rounded shoulders, and sunken-in chests! On the other hand, people of advanced years, by simply straightening their spines and walking more erect, appear 10-30 years younger than they really are! Look around at family, friends, etc. and notice postures of all ages and see what we mean! We enjoy posture watching.

89

One's entire life must be a constant fight to maintain the correct, erect posture, for this then gives your heart and internal organs room to operate more efficiently. Remember, the spine is the fundamental structure of the body. Along with the brain, the spine constitutes the center of the nervous system! All other parts of the body are, so to speak, appendages of the spine. Keep that spinal column straight, keep it flexible and youthful! Good health and longevity depend on a healthy, erect body. Never cross your legs – sit tall with both feet on floor. Stretch up your spine to sit, stand and walk tall. Check your body and posture (best in bathing suit or nude) in full mirror. See where you are on the posture chart – perfect, fair or poor? Start improving from today on!

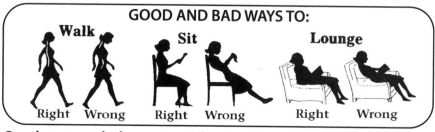

GOOD AND BAD WAYS TO:

Walk — Right   Wrong
Sit — Right   Wrong
Lounge — Right   Wrong

Good posture helps prevent backaches and related problems.

Don't Cross Your Legs – It's Unhealthy

When sitting never cross your legs! Under the knees run two of the largest arteries, called popliteal arteries carrying nourishing blood to the muscles below the knees and to nerves in the feet. You immediately cut down the blood flow to a trickle when you cross your legs.

When the muscles of the legs and knees are not nourished and don't have good circulation, then the extremities stagnate, which can lead to varicose veins and other health problems. Look at the ankles of people age 40 and over who have the habit of crossing their legs. Note the broken veins and capillaries! When the muscles and feet do not get their full supply of blood, the feet become weak and poor circulation sets in. Cold feet usually torment the leg-crosser.

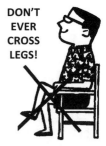

DON'T EVER CROSS LEGS!

A well-known heart specialist was asked, *"When do most people have a heart attack?" He answered, "At a time they are sitting quietly with one leg crossed over the other."* When you sit, plant both feet squarely on floor, or foot stool or box if needed. **Crossing legs puts unnecessary burden on your heart!**

People who are habitual leg-crossers have more acid crystals stored in the feet than those who never cross their legs! Crossing legs is one of the worst postural habits of man. It throws the hips, spine and head off balance and it's the most common cause of chronic backaches, headaches and varicose veins. Be kind to your body – please don't cross your legs. You can break this bad habit.

90

The Dangers of Sitting Too Long

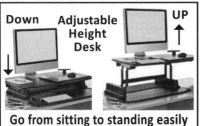

Down Adjustable Height Desk UP

Go from sitting to standing easily with an adjustable stand up desk.

People who sit too long at work, sadly may develop a thrombosis (blood clot) in the deep veins of the calf. If your office work requires you to sit a lot at a computer, *get up, move around every hour or ◀ get an up and down desk.*

WHERE DO YOU STAND?

POSTURE CHART

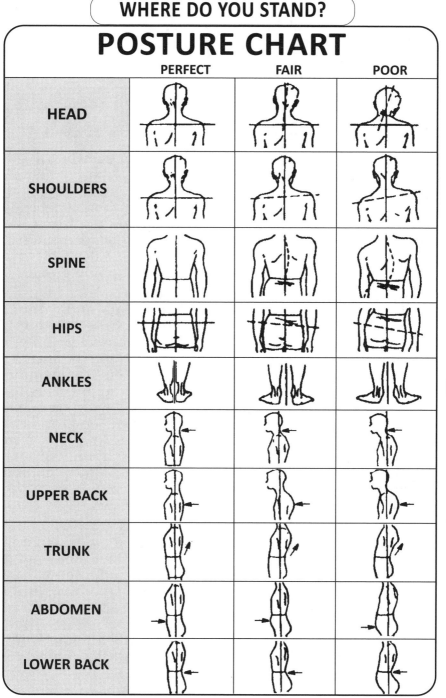

	PERFECT	FAIR	POOR
HEAD			
SHOULDERS			
SPINE			
HIPS			
ANKLES			
NECK			
UPPER BACK			
TRUNK			
ABDOMEN			
LOWER BACK			

91

Your posture carries you through life from your head to your feet. This is your human vehicle and you are truly a miracle! Cherish, respect and protect it by living The Bragg Healthy Lifestyle. – Patricia Bragg

Remember – Your posture can make or break your looks and health!

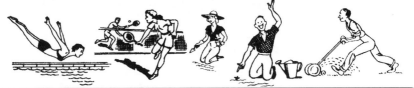

Live The Bragg Healthy Lifestyle
To Enjoy a Lifetime of Super Health!

In a broad sense, "The Bragg Healthy Lifestyle for the Total Person" is the perfect combination of physical, mental, emotional, social and spiritual components. The ability of the individual to function effectively in his environment depends on how smoothly these components function as a whole. Of all the qualities that comprise an integrated personality, a totally healthy, fit body is one of the most desirable . . . so start today to achieve your health and happiness goals!

A person may be said to be totally physically fit if he functions as a total personality with efficiency and without pain or discomfort of any kind. This is to have a Painless, Tireless, Ageless Body, possessing sufficient muscular strength and endurance to maintain a healthy posture and successfully carry on the duties imposed by life and the environment, to meet emergencies satisfactorily and have enough energy for recreation and social obligations after the "work day" has ended. It is to meet the requirements of his environment through possessing the resilience to recover rapidly from fatigue, tension, stress and strain of daily living without the aid of stimulants, drugs or alcohol, and enjoy natural recharging sleep at night and awaken fit and alert in the morning for the challenges of the new fresh day ahead.

Keeping the body totally healthy and fit is not a job for the uninformed or careless person. It requires an understanding of the body and of a healthy lifestyle and then following it for a long, happy lifetime of health! The purpose of "The Bragg Healthy Lifestyle" is to wake up the possibilities within you, rejuvenate your body, mind and soul to total balanced health. It's within your reach, so don't procrastinate, start today! Our hearts go out to touch your heart with nourishing love for your health, happiness and a fulfilled long life!

Patricia and *Paul C. Bragg*

Dear friend, I wish above all things that thou may prosper and be in health as your soul prospers. – 3 John 2

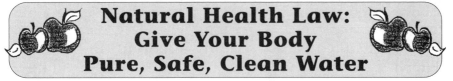

Natural Health Law: Give Your Body Pure, Safe, Clean Water

The body is 75% water, thus drinking purified, steam-distilled (chemical-free) water is important for total health. You should drink 8-10 glasses of water a day. Read our book, *Water – The Shocking Truth* for information on the importance of purified water.

Water – The Body's Vital Lubricant

The body, in its own way, is greased and oiled automatically. The body's basic lubricant is water. It permits organs to slide against each other – as when you bend down. It helps bones to move in their joints. You couldn't bend a knee or elbow without water and it also acts as a shock-absorbing agent to ward off injury from blows. Applied hydraulically in various parts of the body, it is used to build and hold pressures. The eyeball is a good example of this particular function of water. Muscle tone cannot be maintained without adequate water, for the muscles are 75% water. This is another reason why fatigue hits the dehydrated body!

WATER IS KEY TO HEALTH AND ALL BODY FUNCTIONS:

- Elimination
- Circulation
- Digestion
- Bones & Joints
- Muscles
- Metabolism
- Assimilation
- Heart
- Nerves
- Energy
- Sex
- Glands

Drinking 8-10 glasses daily of pure distilled purified water cleanses and water recharges the human batteries! – Paul C. Bragg, N.D., Ph.D.

The problem of Pharmaceuticals in drinking water has been an ongoing health issue for decades (FDA.gov). Polyfluoroalkyl and Perfluoroalkyl (PFASs) exceed federally recommended safety levels in public drinking water supplies. The Agency for Toxic Substances and Disease Registry says some studies have suggested PFASs are associated with developmental health problems in children, decreased fertility and an increased cancer risk.

Water flows through every single part of your body, cleansing and nourishing it. But the wrong kind of water, with inorganic minerals, harmful toxins, chemicals and other contaminants can pollute and clog your body, and gradually stiffening it painfully. – Paul C. Bragg, N.D., Ph.D.

Be Safe – Drink Purified, Distilled Water!

Pure distilled water is vitally important in following The Bragg Healthy Lifestyle. Water is the key to all body functions including: digestion, assimilation, elimination and body circulation, and to bones and joints, muscles, nerves, glands and senses. The right kind of water is one of your best natural protections against all kinds of diseases and infections. It's a vital factor in all the body fluids, tissues, cells, lymph nodes, blood and all glandular secretions. Water holds all nutritive factors in solution, as well as toxins and body wastes, and acts as the main transportation medium throughout the body, for both nutrition and cleansing purposes (page 21).

Since your body is about 75% water and the blood and lymphatic system are over 90% water, it's essential for your health that you drink only pure water that's not saturated with contaminants, inorganic minerals and toxins! This pure water will transport vital nutrients to cells and the waste from cells more efficiently. This allows the body to function correctly and stay healthier!

94

ORGANIC MINERALS: Your minerals must come from an organic source, from something living or that has lived. Humans do not have the same chemistry as plants. Only the living plant has the ability to extract inorganic minerals from the earth and convert them to organic minerals for your body to absorb and utilize them.

INORGANIC MINERALS: The inorganic minerals and toxic chemicals in water can create these problems:

- Arthritis, bone spurs and painful calcified formations in the joints.
- Hardens the liver.
- Kidney and gallstone issues.
- Inorganic minerals and toxic chemicals in water, clog arteries and small capillaries that are needed to feed and nourish your brain with oxygenated blood; result is gradual loss of memory, senility and strokes.

COCKTAIL OF TOXIC CHEMICALS

Chlorine, fluoride, calcium carbonate cadmium, aluminum, trihalomethanes, chloroform, arsenic, copper, lead and unpleasant taste

Tap-Water Average Contents

Distilled water plays vital part in the health treatment of illness, arthritis, etc.
– Dr. Allen E. Banik, author of "The Choice is Clear"

THE 75% WATERY HUMAN

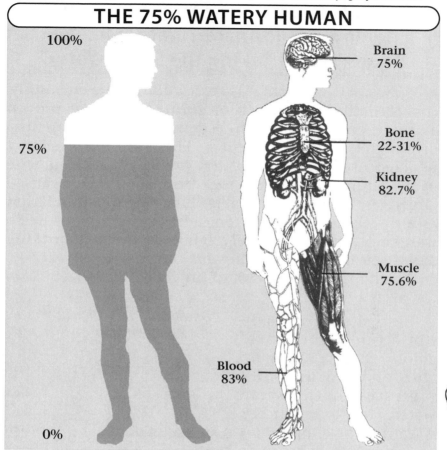

100%

75%

0%

Brain 75%

Bone 22-31%

Kidney 82.7%

Muscle 75.6%

Blood 83%

95

The amount of water in human body, averaging 75%, varies considerably even from one part of the body to another area as shown here. A lean man may hold 75% of his weight in body water, while a woman – because of her larger proportion of adipose tissues – may be only 52% water. The lowering of the water content in the blood is what triggers the hypothalamus, the brain's vital thirst center, to send out its familiar urgent demand for a drink of water! Please obey and drink ample amounts (8 glasses) of purified, distilled water daily. By the time you feel thirsty, you're already dehydrated. – American Running & Fitness Association

WATER PERCENTAGE IN VARIOUS BODY PARTS:

Teeth	10%	Spleen	75.5%
Bones	22-31%	Lungs	80%
Cartilage	55%	Blood	83%
Red blood corpuscles	68.7%	Bile	86%
Liver	71.5%	Plasma	90%
Brain	75%	Lymph	94%
Muscle tissue	75%	Saliva	95.5%

This chart shows why 8-10 glasses of pure water daily is so important.

You Get More Toxic Exposure from Taking a Chlorinated Water Shower Than From Drinking the Same Water!

*Two of the very highly toxic and volatile chemicals, trichloroethylene and chloroform, have been proven as toxic contaminants found in most all municipal drinking U.S. water supplies. The National Academy of Sciences has estimated that hundreds of people die in the United States each year from the cancers caused largely by ingesting water pollutants from inhalation as air pollutants in the home. Inhalation exposure to water pollutants is largely ignored. Recent shocking data indicates that hot showers can liberate about 50% of the chloroform and 80% of the trichloroethylene into the air.

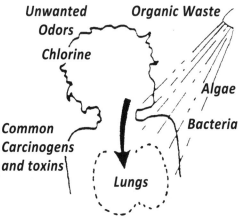

Tests show your body can absorb more toxic chlorine from a 10 minute shower than drinking 8 glasses of the same water. How can that be? A warm shower opens up your pores, causing your skin to act like a sponge. As a result, you not only inhale the toxic chlorine vapors, you absorb them through your skin, directly into your bloodstream – at a toxic rate that is up to 6 times higher than drinking it.

In terms of cumulative damage to your health, showering in chlorinated water is one of the most dangerous risks you take daily. Short-term risks include: eyes, sinus, throat, skin and lung irritation. Long-term risks include: excessive free radical formation (that ages you!), higher vulnerability to genetic mutation and cancer development; and difficulty metabolizing cholesterol that can cause hardened arteries. – *Science News

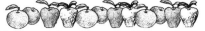

The treatment of diseases should go to the root cause, and most often is found in severe dehydration from lack of sufficient purified distilled water, plus an unhealthy lifestyle! WaterCure.com

Five Hidden Toxic Dangers in Your Shower:

• **Chlorine:** Added to all municipal water supplies, this disinfectant hardens arteries, destroys cells and tissues, irritates skin, sinus conditions and aggravates asthma, allergies and respiratory problems.

• **Chloroform:** This powerful by-product of chlorination causes excessive free radical formation (a cause of accelerated ageing!), normal cells to mutate and cholesterol to form. It's a known carcinogen!

• **DCA (Dichloroacedic acid):** This chlorine by-product alters cholesterol metabolism and has been shown to cause liver cancer in lab animals.

• **MX (toxic chlorinated acid):** Another by-product of chlorination, MX is known to cause genetic mutations that can lead to cancer growth and has been found in all chlorinated water for which it was tested.

• **Cause of bladder and rectal cancer:** Research proved chlorinated water is direct cause of over 9% of U.S. bladder cancers, 15% of rectal cancers and rise in heart disease.

97

Showers, Toxic Chemicals and Chlorine

Water chlorination has been widely used to "purify" water in America starting in 1904. But chlorine's negative effects on health surely outweigh any benefits! "Chlorine is the greatest crippler and killer of modern times! While it prevented epidemics of one disease, it was creating another. Twenty years after the start of chlorinating our drinking water, the present mounting epidemic of heart trouble, cancer and senility began in 1924, and is costing billions." – Dr. Joseph Price, *Coronaries, Cholesterol, Chlorine*

Skin absorption of toxic dangerous contaminants has been gravely underestimated and the ingestion may not constitute the sole primary route of deadly exposure. – Dr. Halina Brown, *American Journal of Public Health*

Read the Bragg Water Book. This book can save your life. Learn why and what kind of water is safest.

We grow healthier in life with safe pure water, healthy foods and love!

Taking long hot showers is a health risk, according to the latest research. Showers – and to a lesser extent baths – lead to a greater exposure to toxic chemicals contained in water supplies than does drinking the water. These toxic chemicals evaporate out of the water and are inhaled. They can also spread through the house and be inhaled by others. People get 6 to 100 times more chemicals by breathing the air while taking showers and baths than they would by drinking the water.
– Ian Anderson, *New Scientist*

A Professor of Water Chemistry at the University of Pittsburgh claims exposure to vaporized chemicals in water through showering, bathing and inhalation is 100 times greater than through drinking the chemicals in water.
– The Nader Report – Troubled Waters on Tap

Don't Gamble – Use a Shower Filter

The most effective method of removing hazards from your shower is the quick and easy installation of a filter on your shower arm. We use a good filter that removes chlorine, lead, mercury, iron, arsenic, hydrogen sulfide, and many other unseen contaminants, such as bacteria, fungi, dirt and sediments. With a 12-18 month life-span, this filter is easily cleaned by backwashing every 2-3 months and is replaceable. So start enjoying safe, chlorine-free showers. It reduces your risk of heart disease and cancer and the strain on your immune system! You may even get rid of long-standing conditions, from sinus and respiratory problems to dry, itchy skin.

Drinking water at correct times maximizes body effectiveness!

- 2 glasses of distilled water in morning helps activate internal organs.
- Glass of water before taking bath/shower helps lower blood pressure.
- Water 2-3 hours before bedtime, helps avoid stroke or heart attack.
- Glass of water with apple cider vinegar 30 minutes before meals, helps improve digestion, gerd and glucose levels. – Gabriel Cousens, M.D.

Man is fully responsible for his nature and his choices. – Jean-Paul Sartre

Pure water is the best drink for a wise man. – Henry David Thoreau

Distilled water plays a vital part in treatment of illnesses. – Dr. Allen E. Banik

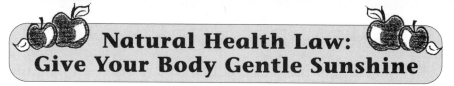

Natural Health Law:
Give Your Body Gentle Sunshine

Enjoy Energy from Gentle Sunbathing

All living things on earth depend on solar energy for their existence. The sun is the primary source of energy. Earth would be a barren, frigid place if it were not for the magic rays of the sun! All things that live, breathe and grow need the energy of the sun. Sun gives us light, and were it not for light, there would be no you or me. Earth would be in darkness and void of life! Mankind gains health, vitality and longevity in the gentle, healing rays of the sun.

People who are deprived of the vital rays of the sun have a pallid look. They are actually dying for want of solar energy! The direct rays of gentle sun on the body supplies vitality and dynamic energy that recharges the human body. **Life-giving sunshine is essential to your health, happiness and longevity.**

Rays of the sun are powerful germicides! As the skin soaks up more of these life-giving rays, it stores enormous amounts of this germ-killing energy and vitamin D. As you bask in the warm, gentle sunshine (not the hot afternoon sun), millions of nerve endings absorb solar energy (*rich in vitamin D3*) and transfer it to your body's nervous system. Gentle sunshine is a soothing tonic, a stimulant and above all, a Great Healer!

Small amounts of gentle sunlight on your skin cells cause them to manufacture vitamin D3. Even as little as 10-15 minutes, 2 to 3 times a week should be enough. Sunscreen can reduce or even shut down the synthesis of vitamin D3, so we recommend exposure to gentle early morning or late afternoon rays without the use of sunscreen.

Sunshine Vitamin D3 – Essential for Health. Analysis of more that 15,000 Americans, with low blood levels of Vitamin D3, were 30% more likely to have high blood pressure, 40% more apt too have high triglycerides, 98% more likely to be diabetic and 129% more apt to be obese. Researchers noted that low Vitamin D3 may also be a culprit for Fibromyalgia, Multiple Sclerosis, Rheumatoid Arthritis and other joint diseases.

Gentle Sunbathing Works Miracles!

When you begin sunbathing, start with short time periods until you condition your body to take more. The best time for beginners to start taking 10 and 15 minute sunbaths is in the early morning sunshine until 10 a.m. or late afternoon sunshine after 3 p.m. Between 11 and 3 we usually avoid stronger, burning rays. Please don't use sunscreen with PABA; the chemicals are harmful.

The cool rays of the sun rejuvenate the skin and also help keep eyes healthy and in focus. Gentle sun is a tonic for frazzled nerves. Its cool rays calm, quiet and soothe the nerves while helping to promote a relaxed feeling. You can combine a nap with a sunbath, you will help refill the body reservoirs with Nerve Force. After gently sunning, pat on some apple cider vinegar (undiluted).

Enjoy God's Sunshine for Super Health

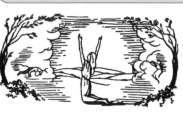

That is why my father and I have always loved basking in precious sunshine and why we made our main home in California, the golden sunshine state. We have an organic farm in Santa Barbara near the ocean where we get benefits of clean air and sunshine. We also lived part-time in Hawaii where we had the Bragg free Exercise Classes at famous Waikiki Beach, 6 days a week. It's fun to exercise in fresh clean ocean air! We enjoyed our students who came from all over the world.

Seek fresh, clean air, gentle sunshine and organic sun-kissed foods, then soon super health will leap out and be yours to treasure throughout a long, ever youthful, fulfilled, happy life!

Sunshine gives energy and life to the earth,
to all plants, trees and all living creatures.

Morning light helps best in the regulation of your body's circadian rhythm and energy balance. Circadian rhythm is the body's physical, mental and behavioral changes that follow a 24-hour cycle.

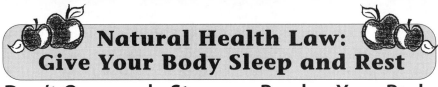

Natural Health Law:
Give Your Body Sleep and Rest

Don't Overwork, Stress or Burden Your Body

Doctor Rest is another Natural Health Law always at your command to help you achieve Supreme Vitality and Health! To us, rest means repose, freedom from activity and quiet tranquility. It means peace of mind and spirit. It means to rest without anxiety or worry! Rest means to refresh and should renew your whole nervous system and your entire body – physically, mentally, and spiritually.

To rest means to allow free circulation (no restrictions) of blood throughout the body, which is important for health. The best rest can only be secured when your body is relaxed and freed from restrictive clothing. Your clothes should be comfortably loose. Are your shoes too tight? Your collar? Your hat? Your stockings? Your watch, belt, undergarments, bra*****? If yes, then you're not resting!

Tension and Relaxation
Create the Heartbeat of Life

As you obey and live by the Laws of Mother Nature you'll automatically earn the right to relax when your body needs relaxation. There is nothing wrong with tension. Tension is part of life. For example – when we walk out onto the platform to lecture before 5,000 people for 2 hours we are bound to feel some tension! Life is movement and movement requires tension as well as release. How is that fact expressed in your body?

You have a miraculous muscle in your chest cavity that is active from the moment it begins to function before birth to the instant of your death. That miracle muscle is your heart. How does it keep going for so many years? Study it closely. Observe exactly how it works. It tenses and then relaxes, tenses and relaxes. Thus it can go on and on and on. There is a great lesson for us here.

****Please read "Dressed To Kill" by S. Singer
on breast cancer and wire bra studies.***

*Women, please cut wires out of bras that hinder your chest circulation.
I prefer not to wear a bra but instead a loose chemise. – Patricia Bragg*

The heart is like life itself. It should be made up of tension and relaxation. To get a task done – whether it is large or small – we must draw upon our Nerve Force reserves. We put an extra push into our efforts and this extra push is tension. If our nerves are healthy and we are working correctly, when the effort of the task is over we should automatically have the feeling of relaxation.

You can't force relaxation any more than you can change the beating of your heart. Relaxation is a feeling, always remember that. It is something that works naturally within your nervous system. Live by Mother Nature's Laws and you will never have to worry about relaxation. This feeling will come to you naturally.

To be able to relax, rest and sleep you must program your day so you have balanced time for work, rest, recreation, exercise and then a good night's sleep. Also, you can't get a good sleep if you overload your stomach! You will enjoy better sleep if you earn it with daily exercise, brisk walking, gardening, etc. We have love and concern for you and love being your health teachers and friends to inspire you to live The Bragg Healthy Lifestyle! Please nourish your body with healthy natural foods, pure distilled water, lots of fresh air, exercise and deep breathing exercises.

Interrupted or Lack of Proper Sleep Can:

- Dramatically weaken your immune system.
- Accelerate tumor growth with severe sleep dysfunctions.
- Cause a pre-diabetic state, making you feel hungry and then you over fuel your body causing obesity.
- Seriously impairs your memory. Even a single night of poor sleep (4-6 hours) can impact ability to think clearly.
- Impairs your performance on physical or mental tasks.
- Can also increase stress-related disorders including: heart disease, stomach ulcers, constipation, mood disorders, personality upsets and depression.

Many people do not earn their rest. Rest must be earned with physical and mental activity, because they go hand in hand. – Paul C. Bragg, N.D., Ph.D.

When your body is completely relaxed then you will experience an inner peace, inner serenity and the true joy of living.

Good Sleep is Cornerstone of Good Health

Eight hours nightly is the optimal amount of sleep for most adults! Science has established that a sleep deficit can have serious, far reaching effects on your health!

Don't Use Toxic Chemicals To Induce Sleep

Sleep is the greatest revitalizer we have, but few people get a long, peaceful and refreshing night's sleep. Most people habitually use stimulants like tobacco, drugs, coffee, tea and other caffeinated drinks which batter tired nerves! People who use these toxic stimulants never have complete rest and relaxation because nerves are always in an excited condition. Sadly millions take some type of drug or alcohol to induce sleep, but this is not true sleep! No one gets restful sleep with sleeping drugs or alcohol. You may drug yourself into unconsciousness, but that very drug will deprive you of a normal, restful, healthy, recharging and satisfying sleep.

Healthy Lifestyle Promotes Sound Sleep

Your nerves are continually irritated when you do not eliminate the toxins from your body. How is it possible to get a good night's rest with irritated nerves? When we faithfully live our Bragg Healthy Lifestyle, exercise, breathe deeply and perform weekly 24-hour fasts, we enjoy and earn sound sleep! We discovered that when our students discard their stimulants and begin a regular fasting program, they too enjoy a more restful, deep sleep.

You will notice as you purify your body that you will be able to relax more readily. You will be able to enjoy naps and you will reap the benefits of a long, restful, night's sleep. Rest is important! The Bible tells us that God appointed one day of rest every week for man. In this wise law, we have ample support for our contention that frequent changes of activity are an important factor in maintaining Super Health. To complement our busy days, we require and enjoy a variety of fun recreational activities. This old adage is true and wise advice to follow: *All work and no play does make Jack and Jill dull and tired.*

Lifestyle Suggestions That Enhance Sleep

- **Avoid stimulants:** caffeine (in coffee, some teas, even green teas, soft drinks, chocolate, sugar) and nicotine (found in cigarettes and other tobacco products).

- **Don't drink alcohol** to "help" you sleep.

- **Have herbal teas** – anise, lemon balm, *Sleepytime*, chamomile (beware some Green Teas have caffeine), or try melatonin, tryptophan (5HTP), valerian, calcium and magnesium supplements; they work miracles.

- **Exercise regularly**, but try to be finished with your workout no sooner than 2 hours prior to bedtime.

- **Avoid foods you may be sensitive to.** Reactions can cause excess congestion, gastrointestinal upset, bloating or gas.

- **Associate your bed with recharging sleep** – it's wise not to sit on it to work or watch TV. *Try a 2" memory foam topper (so comfortable) on your firm mattress.*

- **Don't nap during the day**, if you suffer from insomnia. Remember, earn better sleep by exercise and day activity.

104

Mother Nature Knows What's Best!

We recommend that you return to a more natural way of living in food, clothing, rest and in simplicity of living habits. Strive for harmony with Mother Nature and God. Live as Mother Nature wants. Realize she loves you and you are part of her family. Put yourself in her hands and let her inner wisdom guide you. Mother Nature is eager to inspire and guide you so she can help you perfect your human machine. She can help cleanse, heal and improve your body if you work with her by living a healthier life!

Be good to your body and it will be good to you! Abuse the body and it will punish you with tension, stress, strain, even constipation! Live so that the feeling of relaxation will come to you when it is needed. **Be a friend to yourself! Treat yourself right so you can enjoy a long, healthy and relaxed life. The kingdom of heaven is within.**

Relaxation is a beautiful soothing feeling within your body and mind.

Peace is not a season, it is an important way for a healthy life!

Natural Health Law:
The Miracle of Fasting
Master Key to Internal Purification

If you do a complete water fast for 24 hours each week, soon you will be able to add more fresh fruit and vegetables to your diet. After a fast of 3 or more days, then you can include more foods in a healthy high rate of vibration.

We have faithfully fasted for 24 hours every Monday and the first three days of each month. Wait until you experience this! You will greatly benefit from the inner cleansing and will love the pure, clean, healthy feeling you receive!

Fasting Cleanses, Renews and Rejuvenates

Our bodies have a natural miracle self-cleansing and self-healing system for maintaining a healthy body and our "river of life" – our bloodstream! It's essential we keep our body machinery from head to toes in perfect health and in good working order to maintain life! Fasting is the best detoxifying method! It's also the most effective and safest way to increase elimination of waste buildups and enhance the body's miraculous self-healing and self-repairing process that keeps you healthy.

If you prepare for a fast by eating a cleansing diet for 1 to 2 days, this can greatly help the cleansing process. Fresh salads, fresh vegetables, fruits and their juices, as well as green drinks (alfalfa, barley, chlorophyll, chlorella, spirulina, wheatgrass, etc.) stimulate waste elimination. Fresh foods and juices can literally pick up dead matter from your body and flush it out of the body!

Daily, even on most days during our fasts, our friend Linus Pauling inspired us to take 3,000 mg. of mixed vitamin C powder (C concentrate, acerola, rosehips and bioflavonoids) in liquids. This is a potent antioxidant and flushes out deadly free radicals that produce many harmful effects. Vitamin C also promotes collagen production for new healthy tissues and is especially important if you are detoxifying from prescription drugs or alcohol overload.

Fasting is for internal cleansing, purification to stay healthy and youthful.

Fasting Removes Sludge from Your Pipes

A moderate, well planned distilled water fast (our favorite) or a diluted fresh juice (35% distilled water) fast for beginners can also cleanse your body of excess mucus, old fecal matter, trapped cellular, non-food wastes and helps remove inorganic mineral deposits and sludge from your pipes and joints. Remember your Vinegar drink also helps remove arterial plaque. (For juice fasting and juice combinations, see pages 108-109.)

Fasting works miracles by self-digestion. During a fast your body intuitively will decompose and burn only substances and tissues that are damaged, diseased or unneeded, such as abscesses, tumors, excess fat deposits, excess water and congestive body wastes! Studies show even a short fast (1-3 days) will help accelerate elimination from your liver, kidneys, lungs, bloodstream and skin. Sometimes you will experience dramatic changes (cleansing and healing crises) as accumulated wastes are expelled. With your first fast you may temporarily get a headache, fatigue, body odor, bad breath, coated tongue, mouth sores and even diarrhea as your body is cleaning house! Please be patient with your miracle body!

After a fast your body will begin to self-cleanse and healthfully rebalance! When you follow The Bragg Healthy Lifestyle, your weekly 24-hour fast removes toxins on a regular basis, so they don't accumulate! Your energy levels will amazingly begin to rise – physically, mentally and spiritually. Your creativity will begin to expand. You will feel like a different person – which you are – for now you are being cleansed, purified and reborn. It is truly the Miracle of Fasting.

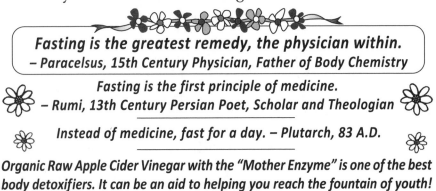

Fasting is the greatest remedy, the physician within.
– Paracelsus, 15th Century Physician, Father of Body Chemistry

Fasting is the first principle of medicine.
– Rumi, 13th Century Persian Poet, Scholar and Theologian

Instead of medicine, fast for a day. – Plutarch, 83 A.D.

Organic Raw Apple Cider Vinegar with the "Mother Enzyme" is one of the best body detoxifiers. It can be an aid to helping you reach the fountain of youth!

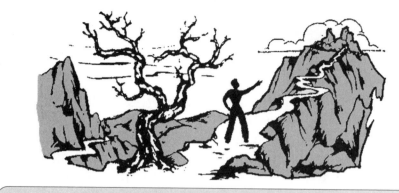

The Trail to Perfect Health

My father and I have always been very loyal to our fasting program. We know what it has done for us, for members of our family, friends, and millions of Bragg health conscious students all over the world. The Bragg Healthy Lifestyle calls for 4 longer fasts a year, along with a weekly 24-or 36-hour fast. We would always fast the first 3 days of every month and all day each Monday.

Remember, it took time for the body to build up toxins, so it takes time to cleanse and unload them! Take your time! You will reap wonderful, priceless, long-lasting health benefits. Please read our book *The Miracle of Fasting* as it gives many more details about the miracle benefits of fasting.

Fasting Brings Miracle Longevity Results

Professor A. E. Crews of Edinburgh University, who studied worms and animals, said: *"Given appropriate and essential conditions, including proper care of the body, Eternal Youth can be a reality in living forms! It's possible, by repeated processes of fasting, to keep an earthworm alive twenty times longer than normal and also proven with animals."* Studies prove life-extending merits of fasting.

In one study, fasting worms every other day caused them to live 50 times as long as usual! The Cornell University studies with rats showed that fasting them systematically increased their life span by 2-3 times!

Fasting is an effective and safe method of detoxifying the body – a technique that wise men have used for centuries to heal the sick. Fasting regularly can help the body heal itself and stay well!
– James Balch, M.D., co-author "Prescription for Nutritional Healing"
"Bragg Books were my conversion to the healthy way."

Juice Fast – Introduction to Water Fast

Fasting has been rediscovered through juice fasting – as a simple, easy means of cleansing and restoring health and vitality. To fast (abstain from food) comes from the Old English word fasten or to hold firm. It's a means to commit oneself to the task of finding inner strength through body, mind and soul cleansing. Throughout history the world's greatest philosophers and sages, including Socrates, Plato, Buddha and Gandhi, and Jesus have enjoyed fasting and preached its benefits.

Although a pure water fast is best, an introductory liquid juice fast can offer people an ideal opportunity to give their intestinal systems restful, cleansing relief from the commercial high fat, high sugar, high salt and high protein fast foods too many Americans exist on.

Organic, raw, live fruit and vegetable juices can be purchased fresh from Health Food Stores. You can also prepare these healthy juices yourself using a juicer or blender. When juice fasting, it's best to dilute juice with $^1/3$ distilled water. This list (next page) gives you many combination ideas. With vegetable and tomato juices try adding Apple Cider Vinegar on non-fast days, even some green powder (barley, chlorella, spirulina, etc.) to create a delicious, nutritious powerful health drink! When using herbs in these drinks, use 1 to 2 fresh leaves.

Paul C. Bragg Introduced Juicing and Smoothies to America

Juicing has come a long way since the first hand operated vegetable-fruit juicers from Europe were available. Before, this juice was pressed by hand using cheesecloth. He introduced his new juice therapy idea, then pineapple juice, then later tomato juice, to the American public. These two juices were erroneously thought to be too acidic. Now, these health beverages have become the favorites of millions. TV's famous *Juicemen* Jay Kordich and Jack LaLanne say Paul Bragg was their early inspiration and mentor! LaLanne also has a great juicer. They both loved living The Bragg Healthy Lifestyle and inspiring millions to health.

Delicious, Powerful Juice or Blender Combinations:

1. Beet, celery, kale and carrots
2. Cabbage, celery and apple
3. Cabbage, cucumber, celery, tomato, kale, spinach and basil
4. Tomato, carrot and celery
5. Carrot, celery, kale, garlic, watercress, blue or goji berries and wheatgrass
6. Grapefruit, orange and lemon
7. Beet, parsley, celery, carrot, mustard greens, cabbage, garlic
8. Beet, celery, kale and carrot
9. Cucumber, carrot and parsley
10. Watercress, apple, cucumber, garlic
11. Asparagus, carrot and apple
12. Carrot, celery, kale, parsley, cabbage, onion and sweet basil
13. Carrot, coconut milk and ginger
14. Carrot, broccoli, lemon, cayenne
15. Carrot, sprouts, kelp, rosemary
16. Apple, carrot, radish and ginger
17. Apple, pineapple and seaweed
18. Apple, papaya and grapes
19. Papaya, blueberries and apple
20. Leafy greens, broccoli, apple
21. Grapes, apple and blueberries
22. Watermelon (alone is best)

Liquefied and Fresh Juiced Foods

The juicer, food processor and blender are great for preparing foods for gentle or bland diets and baby foods. Fibers of fresh fruits and vegetables juiced can be tolerated on most gentle diets. Any raw or cooked fruit or vegetable can be liquefied and added to non-dairy milks – soy, rice, nut, almond, etc., or broth or soups. Fresh juices supercharge your body's health power! You may fortify your liquid meal with barley green, chlorella, soy, spirulina, and vitamin C powder for extra super nutrition!

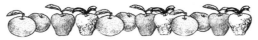

Fasting on raw fruit juices, vegetables broths and herb teas helps aid in a faster recovery from disease. It's an effective body cleanser and rejuvenator.

Let food be your medicine and medicine be your food.
– Hippocrates, 400 B.C.

The body is self-cleansing, self-correcting and self-healing when you give it a chance with a fasting cleanse and living a healthy lifestyle!
– Patricia Bragg, Pioneer Health Crusader and Lifestyle Educator

When fasting, masses of accumulated metabolic wastes and toxins in the body are gathered up and expelled from the body!

BENEFITS FROM THE JOYS OF FASTING

Fasting renews your faith in yourself, your strength and God's strength.
Fasting is easier than any diet.
Fasting is the quickest way to lose weight.
Fasting is adaptable to a busy life.
Fasting gives the body a physiological rest.
Fasting is used successfully in the treatment of many physical illnesses.
Fasting can yield weight losses of up to 10 pounds or more in the first week.
Fasting lowers and normalizes cholesterol, homocysteine, blood pressure levels.
Fasting improves dietary habits.
Fasting increases pleasure eating healthy foods.
Fasting is a calming experience, often relieving tension and insomnia.
Fasting frequently induces feelings of happy euphoria, a natural high.
Fasting is a miracle rejuvenator, helps in slowing the ageing process.
Fasting is a natural stimulant to rejuvenate the growth hormone levels.
Fasting is an energizer, not a debilitator.
Fasting aids the elimination process.
Fasting often results in a more vigorous happy marital relationship.
Fasting can eliminate smoking, drug and drinking addictions.
Fasting is a regulator, educating the body to consume food only as needed.
Fasting saves precious time spent on marketing, preparing and eating.
Fasting rids the body of toxins, giving it an internal shower and cleansing.
Fasting does not deprive the body of essential nutrients.
Fasting can be used to uncover the sources of food allergies.
Fasting is used effectively in schizophrenia and other mental illness treatment.
Fasting under proper supervision can be tolerated easily up to four weeks.
Fasting does not accumulate appetite; hunger pangs disappear in 1-2 days.
Fasting is routine for most of the animal kingdom.

110

Fasting has been a common practice since the beginning of man's existence.
Fasting is practiced in all religions; the Bible alone has 74 references to fasting.
Fasting under proper conditions is absolutely safe.
Fasting is a blessing – "Fasting As A Way Of Life" – Allan Cott, M.D.
Fasting is not starving, it's nature's cure that God has given us. – Patricia Bragg

Dear Health Friend,

This gentle reminder explains the great benefits from "The Miracle of Fasting" that you will enjoy when starting on your weekly 24-hour Bragg Fasting Program for Super Health! It's a precious time of body-mind-soul cleansing and renewal.

On fast days I drink 8-10 glasses of distilled (our favorite) or purified water, (I add 1-2 tsps. organic apple cider vinegar to three of them). If just starting, you may also try herbal teas or try diluted fresh juices with 1/3 distilled water. Every day, even on fast days, add 1 Tbsp. of psyllium husk powder to liquids once daily. It's an extra cleanser and helps normalize weight, cholesterol and blood pressure and helps promote healthy elimination. Fasting is the oldest, most effective healing method known to man. Fasting offers great miraculous blessings from Mother Nature and our Creator. It begins the self-cleansing of the inner-body workings so we can promote our own self-healing.

My father and I wrote the book "The Miracle of Fasting" to share with you the health miracles it can perform in your life. It's all so worthwhile to do. It's an important part of The Bragg Healthy Lifestyle.

With Love,

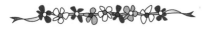

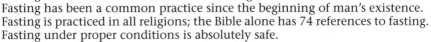

***Paul Bragg's work on fasting and water is one of the great contributions to The Healing Wisdom and The Natural Health Movement in the world today.
– Gabriel Cousens, M.D., author "Conscious Eating" and "Spiritual Nutrition"***

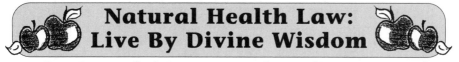
Do Peaceful Prayer and Meditation Daily

"Be still and know that I am God." It is in the peaceful silence of meditation and prayer that you find a higher power than yourself. This power can help guide and direct you towards the healthy goals in life you are seeking.

It is important to set aside a period twice daily – morning and evening – during which time, the mind can go into meditation and prayer to build inner strength. There must be order and clear purpose to your thinking. Silently restate your new goals in life. Remember that you must displace the old, useless and damaging habits of thought with fine, bright, new healthy ideas.

Every constructive thought stimulates the nervous system with great vitality and vigor, and this sustained and powerful activity stimulates the entire body. Through meditation and prayer you are building a strong mind in a healthy strong body and you are opening that inexhaustible reservoir of energy and creative intelligence which lies within each human. Meditation and prayer will help establish equilibrium in mind, body and soul. It infuses you with new energy and expanded awareness, while it instills you with an inner calm and peace. You gain strength to do and to endure – to take the strains and pressures of life in your daily stride.

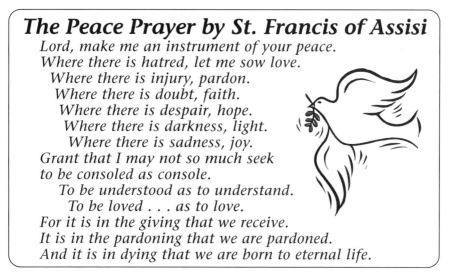

The Peace Prayer by St. Francis of Assisi

Lord, make me an instrument of your peace.
Where there is hatred, let me sow love.
Where there is injury, pardon.
Where there is doubt, faith.
Where there is despair, hope.
Where there is darkness, light.
Where there is sadness, joy.
Grant that I may not so much seek
to be consoled as console.
To be understood as to understand.
To be loved . . . as to love.
For it is in the giving that we receive.
It is in the pardoning that we are pardoned.
And it is in dying that we are born to eternal life.

Daily meditation and prayer gives you a chance to strengthen your resolve to completely follow The Bragg Healthy Lifestyle. Your morning meditation and prayer allows you to plan your day constructively. Your evening meditation and prayer offers opportunity to review your day and evaluate accomplishments and mistakes as you plan how to correct the latter. During this state the body experiences peaceful repose more profound than sleep. Studies have shown the pulse, respiration and metabolism slow down to levels below those ordinarily reached during sleep. People normally feel as refreshed following a session as they would after a nap.

Meditation and Prayer Helps Master Life

Taking inventory of yourself this way is important. You will soon notice a much greater peace, tranquility and health within yourself. Life will flow more easily for you. Annoying events, things and people that used to bother you will no longer have the same effect upon you. This will give you more energy for creative thinking and living.

The release, peace and relaxation that is experienced envelopes the entire day, with a softening effect upon your entire outlook and relations with life and others. The degree of personal involvement in emotional problems is diminished. This is not to say that emotional capacity is weakened! On the contrary, this wellspring is deepened as your inner life achieves greater life balance and stability. Meditation and prayer eliminates the causes of tension in a natural way (not like toxic tranquilizers), as it subtly sharpens the mind, heart and senses. This release from mental tension and physical duress gives a healthy effect on your entire well-being. It helps to build a healthier balance to restore the body's normal rhythm of functions. Millions worldwide benefit from spirituality which gives practical and powerful guidance and love.

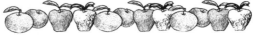

Living in harmony with the universe is living totally alive,
full of vitality, health, joy, inner peace, power, love, and
abundance on every level. – Shakti Gawain

Control Your Negative and Positive Thoughts!

The mind must have a will of iron and always be in command of the body. From this day forward learn how to substitute your thoughts. When negative thoughts – such as, *"I am losing my energy because when you get older you start to lose energy"* – enters your mind, replace it with positive healthy thoughts, say to yourself, *"Age cannot in any way affect my energy. I am ageless!"*

Think of your thoughts as powerful self-talk magnets with the ability to attract (positive) or repel (negative) according to the way used. A majority of people lean either to positive or negative mentalities. The positive phase is constructive and goes for success and positive achievements, while the negative side of life is destructive, leading to futility and failure. It is self-evident it is to our advantage to cultivate a positive, healthy, mental attitude. With patience, persistence and living The Bragg Healthy Lifestyle this can be accomplished!

Always keep in mind that whatever the mind tells the flesh, that is exactly what the flesh is going to believe.

Negative Emotions Bad for Your Health

There are many negative and destructive forms of thought which react in every cell in your body! The strongest is **fear**, and its child, **worry** – along with **depression, anxiety, apprehension, jealousy, ill-will, envy, anger, resentment, vengefulness and self-pity.** All of these negative thoughts bring tension to the body and mind, leading to waste of energy, enervation and also slow or rapid poisoning of the body. **Rage, intense fear and shock are very violent and quickly intoxicate the whole system. Worry and other destructive emotions act slowly but, in the end, have the same destructive effect.** Anger and intense fear stop digestive action, upset the kidneys and the colon causing total body upheaval (diarrhea or constipation, headaches, pains, fever, etc.).

Just by paying attention to breathing, you can access new levels of health, energy and relaxation that will benefit every area of your life.
– Deepak Chopra, M.D. • www.chopra.com

Fear, worry and other destructive habits of thought muddle the mind! A crystal clear mind is needed to reason to your best advantage, enabling you to make sound, healthy decisions! An emotionally, upset clouded mind often makes unwise and unhealthy decisions and might be unable to reach any positive conclusions at all!

Most humans are so full of worry that they believe they can never overcome their miseries. **Worrying about a problem does not solve it – it only makes things worse.** You can literally "worry yourself to death."

Don't Worry, Please Be Happy and Healthy!

The good news is you can control all of these things in short time! Building positive attitude; maintaining a desire for lifelong learning and advancement; and most especially constantly working on reducing self-judgment and criticism, are all highly-effective ways of reducing stress. Daily try laughing out loud (*www.LaughterYoga.org*) and smiling at those around you. Learn to meditate or take relaxing walks; and make sure you assume responsibility for your life and what happens to you and don't blame others. This puts you in control, the Captain of your life, which helps immediately to reduce stress. Added to those efforts, of course, must be a healthy diet, regular exercise, and sufficient sleep. These are all valuable ingredients of achieving good health and once you make it part of your lifestyle, you will become stress-free, heart-healthy and live a longer, stronger, happier, fulfilled life.

How Spiritual Beliefs Impact Healing

Spirituality shapes life's meaning for many people. Inside that meaning lies faith, which brings about trust, positive thinking and hope. Developing and nurturing spiritual values and a deeper sense of purpose can not only keep you healthy and well, but also provide the tools to grow, develop and heal when illness arises.

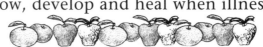

Please be a good, wise, strict, loving, "mother-like captain" to your miracle working body that is carrying you through life!
– Patricia Bragg, Pioneer Health Crusader and Life Coach

Numerous research studies are finding the those who have spiritual practices tend to live longer and that positive beliefs can influence health outcomes. Those who are spiritual tend to have a more positive outlook on life and a better quality of life. Spirituality helps people cope with disease and face the possibility of death with peace. By cultivating a spiritual life, people are able to gain strength, hope and the ability to counteract stress, which most experts believe is at the root of almost all diseases, illnesses and health conditions. Those with a spiritual perspective also tend to believe that disease and illness are the manifestation of negative emotions and thought patterns. Feelings like resentment, criticism, guilt and fear can all lead to an imbalance in the mind and body, creating physical illness that brings with it an opportunity for self-healing. Someone who takes a spiritual approach to illness will often heal once these negative deep-rooted beliefs are addressed and overcome.

Faith and Vision Create Miracles

When you begin to believe you can be what your inner vision tells you that you can become – that's when you're inspired. When you no longer see your weaknesses – but your strengths – then you discover the power and ability to do things you never dreamed of doing before!

During your daily meditation and prayer you must forget your inadequacies and reach inside to find your strength – it's there! See yourself as who you want to be. Paint a vivid picture in your mind. Concentrate on that image in your meditation and prayer times and carry it with you daily. By following The Bragg Healthy Lifestyle, you are working with Mother Nature, powers higher than yourself! You are then living by inspiration, one of the most tremendous forces in this great universe!

Give me the Serenity to accept what cannot be changed;
the Courage to change what can be changed;
and the Wisdom to know the difference.

Whatever occurs in the mind, effects the body and visa versa. Mind and body cannot be considered independently. When the two are out of sync, both emotional and physical stress can erupt. – Hippocrates, 400 B.C.

Those happy, healthy, strong and vigorous people – those people who accomplish greatness – all those of faith, possess a deep spiritual philosophy. They believe that their lives are protected by a Power greater than their own. They believe there is a destiny which guides their lives. Nothing can thwart them! Following the Eternal Laws of Mother Nature they can accomplish great things!

Let Mother Nature and God Inspire You!

We'd like to urge you to ask Mother Nature to inspire you in your prayer and meditations and, while following our Healthy Lifestyle Program, to inspire you in your work, business and home. In Mother Nature you will find a power that will help you reach the heights of more healthy balanced living. Here are more great ingredients for a winning philosophy:

First: During prayer and meditations, dream great dreams and through meditation work to develop a will that translates those dreams into reality for your life.

Second: Find inspiration in some great goal, some worthy cause or real challenge and let someone or something inspire you to see yourself not for what you are, but for what you can become and accomplish in life.

Third: Live by this Bragg Healthy Lifestyle Program, no matter what! Do the greatest good possible within you! Live up to the highest potential that you have! Accomplish those goals which have been set for you by Mother Nature! We know that if you meditate and pray twice to three times daily along these lines and build upon your inner strengths you will win, conquer and triumph with a long, happy, fulfilled life!

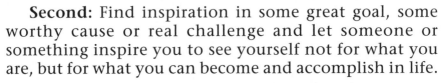

Gloom and Bleakness steals joy, energy and color from your world.
You can't save your life if you don't value it! – "Heart Healthy Living Magazine"

If you truly love Nature, you will find Beauty everywhere. – Vincent Van Gogh

As a single footstep will not make a path on earth, so a single thought will not make a pathway in the mind. To make a deep physical path, we walk again and again. To make a deep spiritual path, we must think over and over the kind of thoughts we wish to dominate our lives. – Henry D. Thoreau

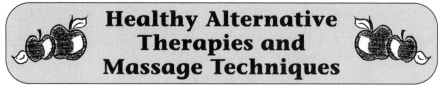

Healthy Alternative Therapies and Massage Techniques

Try Them – They Are Working Miracles!

Explore these wonderful natural methods of healing your body. Over 600 Medical Schools in the U.S. are teaching Healthy Alternative Therapies. Please check their websites. Now seek and choose the best healing techniques for you:

ACUPUNCTURE / ACUPRESSURE: Acupuncture directs and rechannels body energy by inserting hair-thin needles (use only disposable needles) at specific points on the body. It's used for pain, backaches, migraines and general health and body dysfunctions. Used in Asia for centuries, acupuncture is safe, virtually painless and has no side effects! Acupressure is based on the same principles and uses finger pressure and massage rather than needles. Check web: *AcupunctureToday.com*

CHIROPRACTIC: was founded in Davenport, Iowa in 1885 by Daniel David Palmer. There are now many schools in the U.S., and graduates are joining Health Practitioners in all nations of the world to share healing techniques. Chiropractic is popular and the largest U.S. healing profession benefitting literally millions! Treatment involves soft tissue, spinal and body adjustment to free your nervous system of any interferences with normal body functions. Its concern is the functional integrity of the musculoskeletal system. In addition to manual methods, chiropractors use physical therapy modalities, exercise, health and nutritional guidance. Web: *ChiroWeb.com*

COLON HYDROTHERAPY: is a safe and effective practice for supporting detoxification, and improving health and vitality. Contact I-ACT (Int'l Association Colon Hydrotherapy) for a certified colon Hydro-Therapist in your area. Web: *i-act.org*

SKIN BRUSHING: daily is wonderful for circulation, toning, cleansing and healing. Use a dry vegetable brush (never nylon) and brush lightly. Helps purify lymph so it's able to detoxify your blood and tissues. Removes old skin cells, uric acid crystals and toxic wastes that come up through skin's pores. Use loofah sponge for variety in shower or tub.

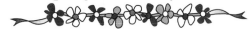

Skin is often called your third kidney because it eliminates toxins from body.

Alternative Health Therapies & Massage Techniques

HOMEOPATHY: In 1796, Dr. Samuel Hahnemann, a German physician, developed homeopathy. Patients are treated with "micro" doses of remedies found in nature to trigger the body's own defenses. This homeopathic principle is a safe and nontoxic remedy and is the #1 alternative therapy in Europe and Britain because it is inexpensive, seldom has any side effects, and usually brings fast results. Web: *HomeopathyCenter.org*

NATUROPATHY: Brought to America by Dr. Benedict Lust, M.D., this treatment uses diet, herbs, homeopathy, fasting, exercise, hydrotherapy, manipulation and sunlight. Practitioners work with your body to restore health naturally. They reject surgery and drugs except as a last resort. Web: *www.Naturopathic.org*

OSTEOPATHY: The first School of Osteopathy was founded in 1892 by Dr. Andrew Taylor Still, M.D. There are now 30 U.S. colleges. Treatment involves soft tissue, spinal and body adjustments that free the nervous system from interferences that can cause illness. Healing by adjustment also includes good nutrition, physical therapies, proper breathing and good posture. Dr. Still's premise: if the body structure is altered or abnormal, then proper body function is altered and can cause pain and illness. Web: *www.AcademyofOsteopathy.org*

REFLEXOLOGY/ZONE THERAPY: Founded by Eunice Ingham, author of *Stories The Feet Can Tell*, inspired by a Bragg Health Crusade when she was 17. Reflexology helps the body and organs by removing crystalline deposits from reflex areas (nerve endings) of feet and hands through deep pressure massage. Primitive reflexology originated in China and Egypt and Native American Indians and Kenyans self-practiced it for centuries. Reflexology activates your body's flow of healing and energy by dislodging deposits. Visit Eunice Ingham and nephew Dwight Byer's website: *www.Reflexology-usa.net*

WATER THERAPY: Soothing detox shower: apply organic olive oil to skin, alternate hot and cold water, every 2-3 minutes. Massage body while under hot, filtered spray. Garden hose massage is great in summer or anytime. Hot detox soak bath (diabetics use warm water) 20 minutes with cup of Epsom salts or apple cider vinegar. This soak helps pull out the toxins by creating an artificial fever cleanse.

My father and I want you to enjoy a fulfilled, healthy, long life.
– Patricia Bragg, Pioneer Health Crusader

Time waits for no one, treasure and protect every moment you have!

ALEXANDER TECHNIQUE: helps end improper use of neuromuscular system, helps bring body posture into balance. Eliminates psycho-physical interferences, helps release long-held tension, and aids in re-establishing muscle tone. For more info see web: *AlexanderTechnique.com*

FELDENKRAIS METHOD: Dr. Moshe Feldenkrais founded this in the late 1940s. This Method leads to improved posture and helps create ease and more efficiency of body movement. This Method is a great stress removal. Web: *Feldenkrais.com*

REIKI: A Japanese form of massage that means "Universal Life Energy." Reiki Massage helps the body to detoxify, then re-balance and heal itself. Discovered in the ancient Sutra manuscripts by Dr. Mikao Usui in Japan 1922. Web: *Reiki.org*

ROLFING: Developed by Ida Rolf in the 1930's in the U.S. Rolfing is also called structural processing and postural release, or structural dynamics. It is based on the concept that distortions (accidents, injuries, falls, etc.) and the effects of gravity on the body cause upsets and long-term stress in the body. Rolfing helps to achieve balance and improved body posture. Methods involve the use of stretching, with gentle deep tissue massage and relaxation techniques to loosen old injuries, break bad movement and posture patterns. Web: *Rolf.org*

TRAGERING: Founded by Dr. Milton Trager, M.D., who was inspired at age 18 by Paul C. Bragg to become a doctor. It is a mind-body learning method that involves gentle shaking and rocking, allowing the body to let go, releasing tensions and lengthening the muscles for more body peace and health. Tragering can do miracle healing where needed in the body frame, muscles and the entire body. Web: *Trager.com*

MASSAGE & AROMATHERAPY: works two ways: the essence (aroma) relaxes, as does healing massages. Essential oils are extracted from flowers, leaves, roots, seeds and barks. These are usually massaged into skin, inhaled or used in a bath to help the body relax, soothe and heal. The oils, used for centuries to treat numerous ailments, are revitalizing and energizing for the body and mind. Example: Tiger balm, MSM, echinacea and arnica help relieve muscle aches. (Avoid skin creams and lotions with mineral oil – it clogs the skin's pores.) Use these natural oils for the skin: almond, avocado, and organic olive oil and mix with aromatic essential oils: rosemary, lavender, rose, jasmine, sandalwood or lemon-balm, etc. – 6 oz. oil and 4 drops of an essential oil. Web: *www.Aromatherapy.com*

MASSAGE – SELF: Paul C. Bragg often said, *"You can be your own best massage therapist, even if you have only one good hand."* Near-miraculous health improvements have been achieved by victims of accidents or strokes in bringing life back to afflicted parts of their own bodies by self-massage and with vibrators. Treatments can be day or night, almost continual. Self-massage also helps achieve relaxation at day's end. Families and friends can learn and exchange massages; it's a wonderful sharing experience. Remember, babies love and thrive with daily massages, start from birth. Family pets also love soothing, healing touch of massages. Web: *RD.com/health/wellness/learn-the-art-of-self-massage*

MASSAGE – SHIATSU: Japanese massage form applies pressure from fingers, hands, elbows and even knees along the same points as acupuncture. Shiatsu originated in Japan and is based on traditional Chinese medicine, and has been widely practiced around the world since 1970s. Shiatsu has been used in Asia for centuries to relieve pain, common ills, muscle stress and to aid lymphatic circulation. See web: *centerpointmn.com/the-benefits-of-shiatsu-massage*

120

MASSAGE – SWEDISH: One of the oldest and the most popular and widely used massage techniques. This deep body massage soothes and promotes healthy circulation and is a great way to loosen and relax tight muscles before and after exercise. See web: *www.MassageDen.com/swedish-massage.shtml*

MASSAGE – SPORTS: An important health support system for professional and amateur athletes. Sports massage improves circulation and mobility to injured tissue, enables athletes to recover more rapidly from myofascial injury, reduces muscle soreness and chronic strain patterns. Soft tissues are freed of trigger points and adhesions, thus contributing to improvement of peak neuromuscular functioning and athletic performance.

Author's Comment: We have personally sampled many of these Alternative Therapies. It's estimated America's health care costs are over $2.6 trillion. It's more important than ever to be responsible for our own health! This includes seeking dedicated holistic health practitioners to keep us well by inspiring us to practice prevention! These Alternative Healing Therapies are also popular and getting results: aromatherapy, Ayurvedic, biofeedback, guided imagery, herbs, hyperbaric oxygen, music, meditation, magnets, saunas, tai chi, Qi gong, Pilates, Rebounder, yoga, etc. Explore them and be open to improving your earthly temple for a healthy, happier, longer life.

Seek and find the best for your body, mind and soul. – Patricia Bragg

Household Cleaning with White Vinegar

We don't endorse white vinegar or dead vinegars for human use, internally or externally! But white vinegar is great for a variety of household, workshop and pet chores, and is safe, effective and an inexpensive household cleaner, deodorizer and disinfectant; which replaces commercial household cleaners that are full of chemicals and additives harmful to you and Mother Nature! Please remember: use only the healthiest – raw, organic apple cider vinegar (*with "mother enzyme"*) for all human consumption and for skin, hair and your pets.

WHITE VINEGAR USES FOR CLEANING KITCHEN

- **Appliances and Counter tops:** clean and disinfect with a white vinegar-dampened sponge or cloth.
- **Greasy Areas:** mix $1/4$ cup white vinegar with 2 cups hot water and add 1 to 2 dashes of biodegradable liquid soap. (Keep mixture in handy, labeled spray bottle.)
- **Sponges and Dish Rags:** disinfect and deodorize by soaking overnight in 1 quart hot water with $1/4$ cup vinegar.
- **Chopping and Bread Boards:** wipe down with full-strength white vinegar to disinfect – leave overnight; or sprinkle with baking soda before spraying with vinegar, wait an hour before wiping clean, then rinse with water.

- **Pots, Pans, Cups:** clean and polish with paste of baking soda and white vinegar. Removes stubborn stuck-on food, stains with 50/50 vinegar-water soak.
- **Glass and China:** stop spotting by mixing $1/2$ cup white vinegar in dishwater, or by placing 1 cup vinegar on bottom rack of dishwasher before starting wash.
- **Drains and Pipes:** keep fresh-smelling and free-flowing with $1/3$ cup of baking soda followed by a cup of white vinegar. Cover drain opening with plate for an hour or longer before flushing through with cold water.
- **Garbage Disposals:** keep clean by grinding up frozen white vinegar ice cubes once weekly (80/20 vinegar-water solution to make cleansing ice cubes).

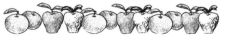

Wash vegetables, salad greens and fruits in a vinegar wash ($1/3$ cup white vinegar to 2 to 3 cups water) to help remove any sprays, etc.

WHITE VINEGAR USES FOR THE BATHROOM

- **Chrome and Stainless Steel:** straight white vinegar will disinfect and polish fixtures; apply with sponge, then buff with soft cloth. Soak grimy shower heads.

- **Garbage Pails:** disinfect with a warm water and white vinegar solution. Let set for an hour or overnight.

- **Shower Curtains:** put through washer rinse cycle with 1 to 2 cups white vinegar. Spray occasionally with 50/50 vinegar-water solution, helps prevent mold.

- **Sink, Tub and Shower:** spray with 80/20 vinegar-water mixture, leave 10 minutes, then scrub and rinse.

- **Toilet Bowl:** use $1/2$ cup straight white vinegar, let stand hour or overnight and flush. For bad stains, follow vinegar with biodegradable cleanser, after 2 hours brush and flush. If stains persist use Clorox bleach ($1/2$ cup) overnight.

WHITE VINEGAR USES FOR LAUNDRY ROOM

- **Washer Tub and Hoses:** remove soap accumulations by running machine for full cycle with pint of white vinegar.

- **New Clothes, Linens, etc:** to remove manufacturing chemicals and new smell odors, add 1 to 2 cups white vinegar to first wash before using. (Never use toxic perfume soaps.)

- **Perspiration Odors (clothes, socks, etc.) and Stained Clothes:** soak overnight in $1/4$ cup vinegar and enough water to cover or soak in washer or pan, then wash in morning.

- **Clothes Final Rinse Cycle:** to help remove static and lint add $1/3$ cup white vinegar.

- **To Soften and Disinfect Fabric, Clothes, Diapers, etc:** add $1/4$ cup white vinegar to most laundry loads. (Don't ever use toxic fabric softeners, they irritate your skin.)

- **Fruit and Grass Stains:** dab with straight white vinegar within 24 hours to safely remove most stains and spots.

- **Musty Smells:** to remove odor and freshen clean cotton clothes just sprinkle with white vinegar and press.

- **Irons:** to eliminate mineral deposits, fill iron with white vinegar and allow to steam on rag, then fill with distilled water and turn upside down to let water drain out. To remove burn stains, mix one part salt with one part vinegar in heated small aluminum pan. Use this mix to polish iron as you would silver.

Do not mix bleach and vinegar. These two common cleaning agents should never be used at the same time, as it will emit toxic vapors. – VinegarTips.com

VINEGAR USES FOR FLOORS, WALLS & FURNITURE

- **Floors:** sponge mop, 1 cup white vinegar in bucket warm water. Also removes residue left by toxic cleaners.
- **Grout:** soak with vinegar, buff with old toothbrush.
- **Carpets:** light stains are extracted by using a mix of 2 Tbsps. salt and 1/2 cup white vinegar, rub the paste mix into carpet and allow to dry before vacuuming.
- **Furniture:** remove cloudy look and brighten by rubbing with mixture of 1 Tbsp. white vinegar in quart warm water, then buff with a soft cloth. Helps remove white rings and scratches from wood tables with a mix of 50/50 vinegar and olive oil or use only olive oil, it works!
- **Vinyl Surfaces:** wipe down with 2 Tbsps. liquid soap and 1/2 cup white vinegar, then water rinse and dry.
- **Toys:** Clean and disinfect with a light spray of vinegar (50/50 vinegar-water solution) and brush or wipe clean.
- **Air Freshener:** mask kitchen odors by simmering a pot of water with 1/2 cup white vinegar.
- **Windows** (also shower doors): spray 50/50 vinegar-water mix, then wipe clean with squeegee. (Great for eye glasses.)

WHITE VINEGAR USES FOR OUTSIDE

- **Ants:** spray equal parts vinegar and water on areas where ant invasions start and surrounding areas. (Chili powder and salt also work.) Vinegar works as a non-toxic pesticide.
- **Car & Car Windows:** keep frost-free with coating solution of 50/50 white vinegar to water. Also helps dissolve old decals and chewing gum with straight white vinegar.
- **Paint Brushes:** to soften soak in boiling white vinegar. Pan of vinegar helps absorb new paint odor and toxic vapors!
- **Fresh-Cut Flowers:** to preserve add 2 tsps. vinegar to quart warm water in vase. Cut ends and renew water every 3 days.
- **Unwanted Grass & Weeds:** pour on straight vinegar.

Create your own ginger-citrus vinegar cleaner by infusing white distilled vinegar with fruit peels for 2-3 weeks. See web: VinegarTips.com

---

Ensure easy upkeep for a beautiful and healthy garden with Vinegar! Environmentally-friendly Vinegar is useful in general garden upkeep and plant and flower maintenance as well as.

Vinegar is an essential home-cleaning item for a beautiful house!

- **Melt Icy Driveways:** A solution of dolomite lime (available at gardening stores) and white vinegar is less damaging to the roads and environment than salt and doesn't harm vehicles.

- **Cut the Rust:** To free a rusted or corroded screw or bolt, soak in white vinegar.

- **Bumper and Label Stickers:** sponge with white vinegar repeatedly until wet. In a few minutes it should peel off easily. *Caution* – test on small area not to damage paint, books, etc.

- **Fireplaces:** Wash with 50/50 water and vinegar to remove blackened soot on walls and glass front doors.

- **Gold Jewelry Cleaner:** Use $1/2$ cup white vinegar. Try soaking gold jewelry in vinegar for 15 minutes. Remove, dry with soft cloth.

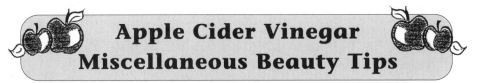

Apple Cider Vinegar
Miscellaneous Beauty Tips

- **Thick & Shiny Hair:** Add 2 Tbsps. apple cider vinegar to 2 cups warm water. Use as a final rinse (see recipe page 44).

- **Rosy Glow:** Apply apple cider vinegar directly to face. Skin will have youthful glow and feel soft and radiant.

- **Soft Feet:** Fill dishpan with warm water and $1/2$ cup ACV. Soak feet 10 minutes or longer. Feet will become softer.

- **Smooth Hands:** Dab apple cider vinegar on hands and arms, helps lighten age spots and skin will feel softer.

- **Alleviate age spots:** Dab age spots, or liver spots, with apple cider vinegar every night before you go to sleep. Do not wash off vinegar. If you feel a stinging sensation, dilute vinegar with water. Wash off in the morning.

- **Dentures:** Dentists advise removing dentures overnight to allow mouth to rest. Soak dentures overnight in ACV, then in morning brush any tartar off with toothbrush. It's natural and non-toxic and less costly than denture-cleaning toxic solution. Apple cider vinegar has antifungal properties and will help fight off Candida from dentures.

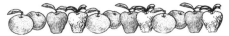

Liven up lettuce and greens – put stems in cold water and ACV.

Add ACV when cooking cabbage to prevent odor in house.

ACV Uses for Pets

- **Good Pet Health:** Add 1 tsp. organic ACV to your pet's water bowl. This is food for your pet's coat and for cleansing inner body of toxins. The natural ACV acidity helps regulate digestion and pectin helps keep their intestines healthier.

- **Fat-Buster for Cats and Dogs:** Please help your pets stay healthy by adding 1 tsp. ACV to drinking water twice a day to help dissolve fats. ACV is great way to help keep pets fit and trim gradually and safely.

- **Bath Time:** After shampooing dog or cat add 2 Tbsps. ACV to pitcher of warm rinse water, pour over pet and watch remaining soap and dead fleas come out.

- **Fight Fleas, Ticks and Mites:** Flea collars and sprays are toxic! Instead use apple cider vinegar (or see tip below). Drop 1 tsp. ACV in water bowl, dab on skin and swab ears if mites are present.

- **Stop Pet Rash and Itch:** For neck and face areas, rear ends and other irritated areas spray or pat on ACV twice daily.

- **Horse Care:** Spruce up horses' coat by adding 1/2 cup ACV to 1 quart water. Use this mixture in spray bottle to apply to horse's coat before showing. Pour 1/4 cup of ACV onto a horse's regular grain feed once a day to deter pesky flies.

WHITE VINEGAR USES FOR PETS:

- **Litter Boxes:** Spritz bottom of litter pan with white vinegar to clean and deodorize. Let pan soak if urine buildup, then rinse clean. On spraying marking areas, clean, then dab on white vinegar to discourage.

- **Skunk Odor:** Spray or dab white vinegar on area, watch smells disappear and it's chemical free!

- **Clean Fish Tank:** Mix white vinegar with your water as you clean the tank. Rinse well, repeat if needed. You'll enjoy clear, clean glass tank and healthier fish.

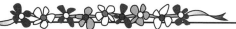

Learning is finding out what you already knew.
Doing is demonstrating that you know it!
Teaching is reminding others that they know it
just as well as you! You are all learners,
doers and teachers! – Richard Bach

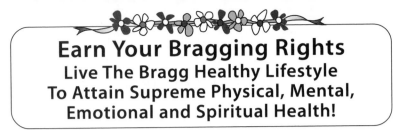

Earn Your Bragging Rights

Live The Bragg Healthy Lifestyle To Attain Supreme Physical, Mental, Emotional and Spiritual Health!

With your new awareness, understanding and sincere commitment of how to live The Bragg Healthy Lifestyle!

God bless you and your family and may He give you the strength, the courage and the patience to win your battle to re-enter the Healthy Garden of Eden while you are still living here on Earth with more years to enjoy it all!

With Blessings of Health, Peace, Joy and Love,

Paul and *Patricia*

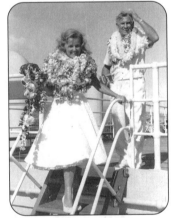

Health Crusaders Paul C. Bragg and daughter Patricia traveled the world spreading health, inspiring millions to renew and revitalize their health.

The Bragg books are written to inspire and guide you to health, fitness and longevity. Remember, the book you don't read won't help. So please reread Bragg Books and live The Bragg Healthy Lifestyle to enjoy a healthy fulfilled life!

I never suspected that I would have to learn how to live – that there were specific disciplines and ways of seeing the world that I had to master before I could awaken to a simple, healthy, happy, uncomplicated life.– Dan Millman, author "The Way of the Peaceful Warrior" • peacefulwarrior.com A Bragg fan and admirer since his Stanford University coaching days.

A truly good book teaches me better than to just read it, I must soon lay it down and commence living in its wisdom. What I began by reading, I must finish by acting! – Henry David Thoreau

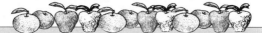

Praises for Apple Cider Vinegar & The Bragg Healthy Lifestyle

I was having 15 to 20 hot flashes a day and tried just about everything including homeopathy and acupuncture with no results. A few weeks ago a friend told me about apple cider vinegar for menopause discomforts so I tried it right away and what a gift from heaven! After a couple days of taking 3 to 4 vinegar drinks a day of the apple cider vinegar all my hot flashes are gone! This is too good to be true! Thank you for this miracle! – Maria Rodriguez, California

---

Apple Cider Vinegar – Miracle Health System is the icing on the cake – a must-read book! I had always heard about ACV . . . everyone in the world should be drinking this on a daily basis! The book is extremely informative and delightful to read. It answers all your questions and then some. Patricia and Paul's books have changed my life!!! – Dr. Steven Gibb

---

Paul Bragg inspired me many years ago with *Miracle of Fasting* and his philosophy on health. His daughter Patricia is a testament to the ageless value of living The Bragg Healthy Lifestyle. – Jay Robb, author, *The Fruit Flush*

I was diagnosed with diabetes and had high sugar levels. Within only 6 months, I was insulin free! I am healthier now than I have been for the past 15 years. My wife, three young children and I are now all healthy vegetarians and living the Bragg Healthy Lifestyle. The results have been amazing! We all thank You. – Dennis Urbans, Australia

---

I read your book on Apple Cider Vinegar and now I take it daily. After passing the book on to my mom, she started using it and the pain in her shoulder that had been waking her up for years has vanished! We both thank you. – Catherine Cox, Toronto, Canada

---

After using organic apple cider vinegar and honey mix for two weeks along with the health ideas expressed in your *Apple Cider Vinegar* Book, I have noticed remarkable improvement in my joints. It's almost unbelievable how fast this has helped! Thank You.
– Tyrone Robinson, Missouri

The Bragg Healthy Lifestyle, vinegar drink and brisk walking (3x daily) 20 minutes after meals, helped eliminate my diabetes! My whole body, circulation, feet, eyes have all improved. Thank you, may God continue to bless your Crusade. – John Risk, California

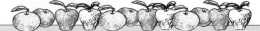

Praises for Apple Cider Vinegar & The Bragg Healthy Lifestyle

I recently had food poisoning and was constantly vomiting and had diarrhea for days. I tried everything I could find over the counter. Nothing worked. Then apple cider vinegar was recommended to me by a family member. What a miracle! Instantly I could feel it working. I am a customer for life! Thanks. – Crystal Escamilla, New Mexico

I recently read the Bragg book *Apple Cider Vinegar Miracle Health System*. I am a believer!! I will be looking for the rest of your books. It is the most uplifting, honest, easy to read, informative book ever on health, nutrition and a positive mind, thank you. – Robyn Scollo, NY

I found your *Apple Cider Vinegar Book* in a health food store. I bought it, read it and gave copies to several friends, including my doctor. I am faithfully following The Bragg Healthy Lifestyle. I can honestly say that all of your Health Books have benefitted me!
– Reiner Rothe, Vancouver, Canada

Thank you Patricia for our first meeting in London in 1968. You gave me your *Fasting Book*, it got me exercising, brisk walking and eating more wisely. You were a blessing God-sent. – Reverend Billy Graham

I use Organic Apple Cider Vinegar for leg cramps. Also ACV is the ONLY thing I have found in 15 years that calmed my restless-leg-syndrome. Thanks so much! – Audra Lynn Weathers, South Carolina

Results with Bragg Healthy Lifestyle and Vinegar are miraculous! I got rid of a constant cold and mucus. I feel so good, energetic and healthy again. Thank You! – Nestor R. Villagra, Toronto, Canada

I've stopped the pain of a burn with full-strength ACV. I also use it to zap occasional skin break-outs (yes, even at 40!) on my face. It has kept my Rosacea flare-ups away. – Jill Hider Peters, Ohio

Many Blessings to you. I have been using ACV with great success. My sinuses and lungs have cleared up. No more excess mucus, my head is clear, I've lost weight and feel naturally more happy. ACV is more effective than any combination of any herbs I have used in the past and is so affordable. Everyone should add this healthy remedy to their diet. It will add joy and years to anyone's life.
– Mahashakti Das, California

PATRICIA & PAUL C. BRAGG, N.D., Ph.D.
Dynamic Daughter & Father are World Health Crusaders

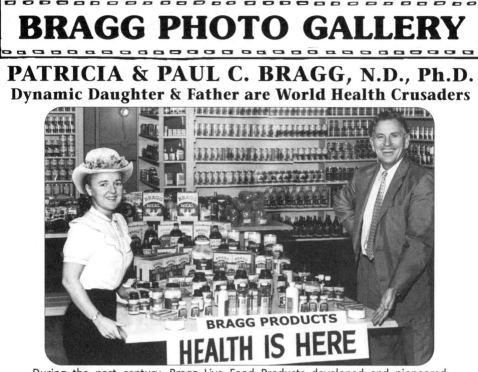

BRAGG PRODUCTS
HEALTH IS HERE

During the past century, Bragg Live Food Products developed and pioneered the very first line of Health Foods, from vitamins and minerals to organic nuts, seeds, and sun-dried fruits. This included over 365 health products, – *"one for each day of the year!"* says daughter Patricia Bragg.

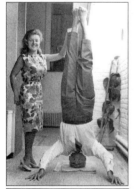

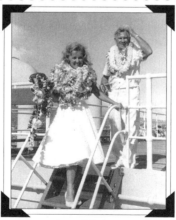

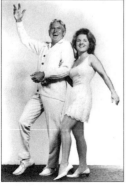

"Thanks for The Bragg Healthy Lifestyle that you shared with me and you are sharing with millions of others worldwide."
– John Gray, Ph.D., author

Picture from
People Magazine August, 1975.

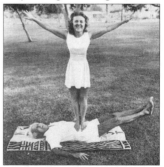

Patricia and father, Paul on world trip in 1950's, during stop in Tahiti.

"You have recharged me with joy, hope, love and encouragement, which poured from your words. I am now fasting and using ACV. You have certainly improved my life!"
– Marie Furia, New Jersey

Patricia Bragg stands on her father's stomach. Paul's stomach muscles are so strong he can lift Patricia up and down!

129

PAUL C. BRAGG, N.D., Ph.D. HEALTH CRUSADER

Life Extension Specialist and Originator of Health Food Stores

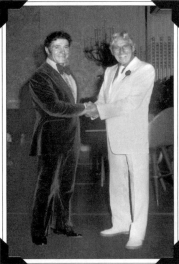

I have experienced a beautiful, remarkable, spiritual and physical awakening since reading Bragg Health Books. I'll never be the same again.
– Sandy Tuttle, Ohio

> ❀ **With every new day comes new strength and new thoughts.** ❀
> *– Eleanor Roosevelt*

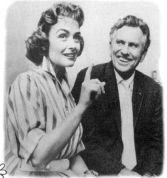

Actress Donna Reed saying "Health First" with Paul C. Bragg.

Dr. Paul C. Bragg (right) Creator Health Food Stores, Pioneer Life Extension Specialist, with his prize student Jack LaLanne. Paul started him on the royal road to health over 85 years ago!

Paul C. Bragg spent much of his time at the Hollywood Studios meeting with top Stars and motion picture industry executives, giving health lectures and private consultations. Dr. Paul C. Bragg was Hollywood's first highly respected, health, fitness and nutrition advisor to the Stars.

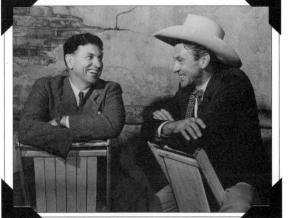

Paul C. Bragg with Gary Cooper, famous American film actor, best known for his many Western films.

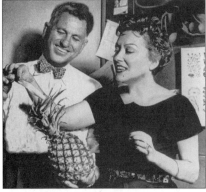

Paul C. Bragg with the famous Hollywood Actress Gloria Swanson, who was leading star in 20s, 30s and 40s. Gloria became a Bragg Health Devotee at 18 and she often would Health Crusade with Bragg during the 1950s.

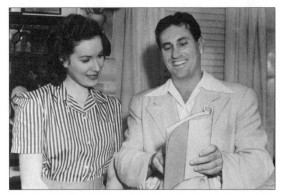

Maureen O'Hara and Paul C. Bragg. This Irish film actress and singer was best noted for playing in "Miracle on 34th Street" and "The Quiet Man."

PAUL C. BRAGG, N.D., Ph.D. STAYING HEALTHY & FIT

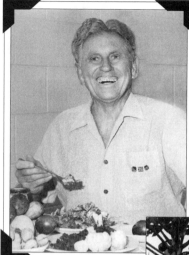

I'd like to thank you for teaching me how to take control of my health! I lost 55 pounds and I feel "great!" Bragg books have showed me vitality, happiness and being close to Mother Nature. You both are real "Crusaders for Health for the World." Thanks!
– Leonard Amato

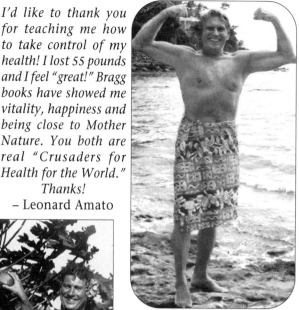

Dr. Paul C. Bragg and daughter Patricia were my early guiding inspiration to my health career.
– Jeffery Bland, Ph.D., Famous Food Scientist

The best thing about the future is that it only comes one day at a time.
– Abraham Lincoln

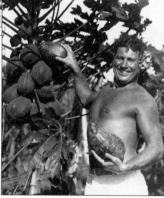

Paul C. Bragg in Tahiti 1920's gathering tropical papaya fruit.

Paul C. Bragg owes his powerful body and superb health to living exclusively on live, vital, healthy, organic rich foods.

Dear Friends – you cannot know how greatly you have impacted my life and some of my friends! We love your Bragg Health Books, teachings and products and are now living healthier, happier lives. Thanks!
– Winnie Brown, Arizona

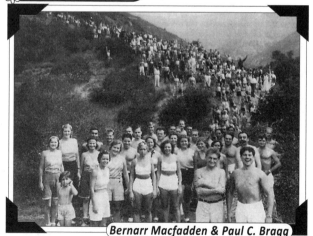

Bernarr Macfadden & Paul C. Bragg

A thousand happy Bragg Health Students enjoy hiking, exercise and fresh air on the trail to Mount Hollywood (above Griffith Observatory) in beautiful California, summer of 1932.

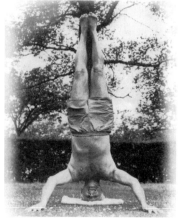

Paul C. Bragg exercising Regent's Park, London.

PHOTO GALLERY

PAUL & PATRICIA BRAGG

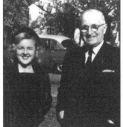

Patricia with 33rd President Harry S. Truman at his home in Independence, Missouri.

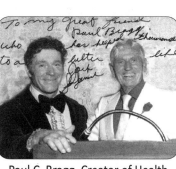

Paul C. Bragg, Creator of Health Food Stores, with his prize student Jack LaLanne, who thanks Bragg for saving his life at 15.

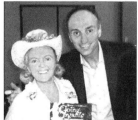

Patrica Bragg with Dr. Jeffrey Smith. He is leader in getting GMO's out of US foods. See GMO video by Jeffrey Smith and narrated by Lisa Oz (Dr. Oz's wife) on web: *GeneticRouletteMovie.com*

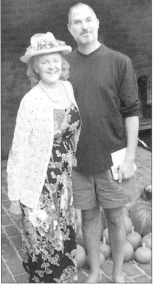

Patricia visiting with Steve Jobs at his home in Palo Alto during the Thanksgiving Holidays.

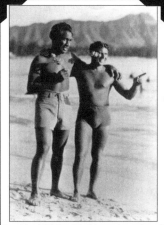

Paul in 1920 with his swimming & surfing friend, Duke Kahanamoku, Waikiki Beach, Diamond Head.

"I've been reading Bragg Books since high school. I'm thankful for the Bragg Healthy Lifestyle and admire their Health Crusading for a healthier, happier world."
– Steve Jobs, Creator –
Apple Computer

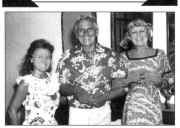

Patricia, Paul C. Bragg and Mrs. Duke (Nadine) Kahanamoku. (Nadine is Patricia's Godmother).

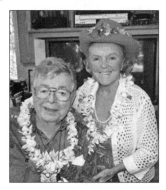

Dr. Earl Bakken with Patricia. He's famous for inventing the first Transistor Pacemaker. His firm Medtronic, developed it and a Resuscitator for fixing ailing hearts that have and are saving thousands of lives. Dr. Bakken lived in Hawaii.

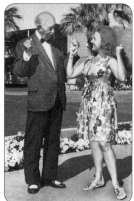

*"I cannot remember a time when the Golden Rule * was not my motto and precept, the torch that guided my footsteps."* – J.C. Penney

*The Golden Rule: Do unto others as you would have them do unto you.

J.C. Penney & Patricia → exercising. They walked often in Palm Springs when he and his wife visited in the winter to enjoy the warm desert sunshine.

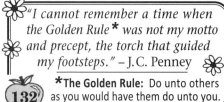

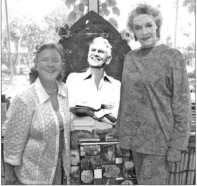

Patricia with friend Actress Jane Russell. Famous Hollywood Star of 40s to 60s.

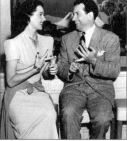

Jane Wyatt learning about health with Paul C. Bragg.

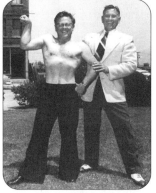

Mickey Rooney with Paul. Rooney was an American film actor and entertainer. He won multiple awards and had one of the longest careers of any actor to age 93!

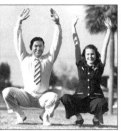

Paul C. Bragg exercising with Actress Helen Parrish.

"Thank you Paul & Patricia Bragg for my simple, easy-to-follow Healthy Lifestyle. You make my days healthy!" – Clint Eastwood, Academy Award Winning Film Producer, Director, Actor and Bragg follower for over 65 years.

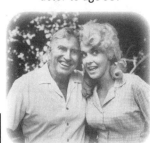

Paul C. Bragg and Donna Douglas, one of Hollywood's most beautiful and talented health advocates. She played the part of "Elly-May" in the *Beverly Hillbillies*, which became one of the longest-running series in television history and was the #1 show in America in its first 2 years.

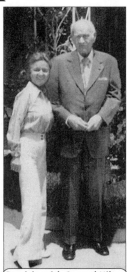

Patricia with Conrad Hilton

← Hotel founder, Conrad Hilton with Patricia Bragg, his Healthy Lifestyle Teacher. *"I wouldn't be alive today if it wasn't for the Braggs and their Bragg Healthy Lifestyle!"* – Conrad Hilton

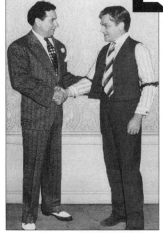

Paul C. Bragg with James Cagney, American film actor. He won major awards for wide variety of roles. The American Film Institute ranked Cagney 8th among the Greatest Male Hollywood Stars of All Time.

"Thank you for your website. What a wealth of info to learn about how to live and eat healthy. Many Blessings!" – Michel & Mary, California

133

PHOTO GALLERY

PAUL C. BRAGG, N.D., Ph.D. PROMOTES HEALTH & FITNESS!

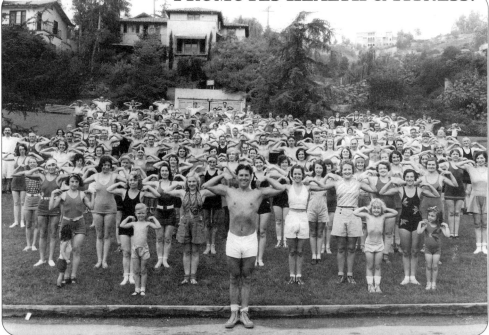

Paul C. Bragg leading an exercise class in Griffith Park, Hollywood, CA – circa 1920s.

Bragg Healthy Lifestyle works Miracles! – Jack LaLanne

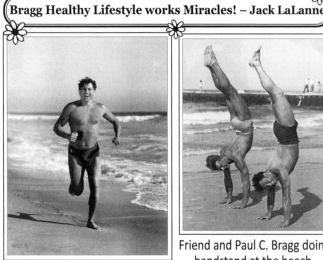

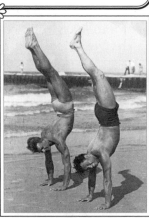

Friend and Paul C. Bragg doing handstand at the beach.

Paul running on Coney Island, New York, where he was a member of the Coney Island Polar Bear Club, known for Cold Water Swimming, 1930s.

TV Hulk Actor Lou Ferrigno gives thanks to Bragg Books. Lou went from puny to become Super Hulk! ➡

Patricia with Lou and wife Carla at Elaine LaLanne's 90th Birthday Party.

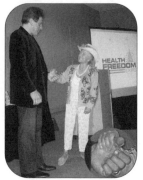

"I lost 102 lbs. with The Bragg Healthy Lifestyle and I have kept it off for over 15 years, staying away from white flour, sugar and other processed foods." – Dee McCaffrey, Chemist & Diet Counselor, Tempe, AZ

Lou & Patricia in Chicago Health Freedom Expo.

PATRICIA CONTINUING BRAGG HEALTH CRUSADE!

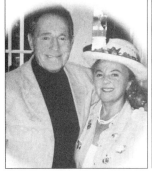

Jack LaLanne with Patricia.

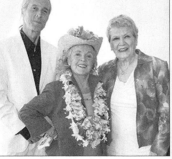

Jon & Elaine LaLanne with Patricia.

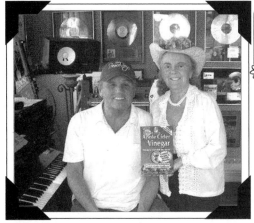

Patricia in studio with famous Beach Boy Bruce Johnston, Bragg follower over 40 years. He played for her their latest records.

Mother Nature Loves US!

Patricia Bragg with Bill Galt inspired by Bragg Books, he founded Good Earth Restaurants.

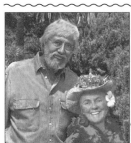

Patricia with Jean-Michel Cousteau Ocean Explorer & Environmentalist. OceanFutures.org

Enjoy a Lifetime of Radiant Health

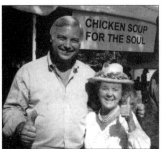

Patricia with Jack Canfield, Bragg follower, Motivational Speaker and Co-Producer of *Chicken Soup For The Soul*.

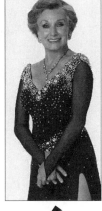

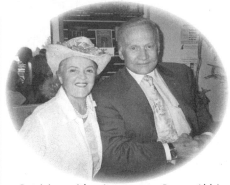

Patricia with Astronaut Buzz Aldrin, celebrating over 50 years since pilot of Apollo 11 first landed on the moon.

Famous Hollywood Actress Cloris Leachman, ardent health follower who sparkled with health and vitality said, *"The Miracle of Fasting Book is a miracle . . . it cured my asthma, my years of arthritis and many other health problems. I praise Paul and Patricia daily for their Health Crusading!"*

PAUL & PATRICIA BRAGG HEALTH CRUSADING

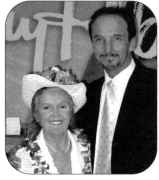

Patricia with Jay Robb.

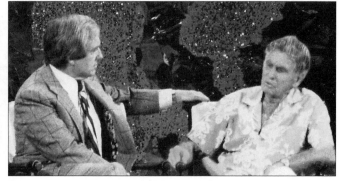

Paul C. Bragg on the Merv Griffin Show, 1976.

Paul Bragg inspired me many years ago with The Miracle of Fasting Book and his pioneering philosophy on health. His daughter Patricia is a testament to the ageless value of living The Bragg Healthy Lifestyle. – Jay Robb, author of *The Fruit Flush*

During the many years Patricia worked with her father, she was right beside him, assisting him on Bragg Health Crusades worldwide. They were a great team, when you looked at them, you would see only two people headed in the same healthy direction!

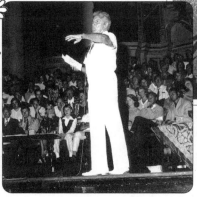

I am a big fan of Paul Bragg. I fast and follow The Bragg Healthy Lifestyle daily. The world and I are blessed with the health teachings of Paul and Patricia Bragg!
– Tony Robbins • *TonyRobbins.com*

❀ **Dream big, think big and enjoy the many miracles.** ❀

Paul & Daughter Patricia, Royal Hawaiian, Honolulu.

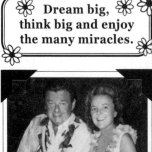

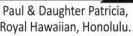

Paul – London Bragg Health Crusade.

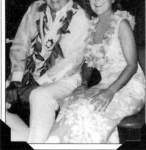

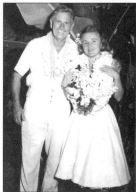

Actor Arthur Godfrey with Patricia, in Honolulu celebrating his 79th birthday.

Health Crusaders Paul C. Bragg and daughter Patricia traveled the world spreading health, inspiring millions to renew and revitalize their health.
Bragg Mottos:
3 John 2 and Genesis 6:3

100 YEAR HISTORY OF BRAGG HEALTH BOOKS & PRODUCTS

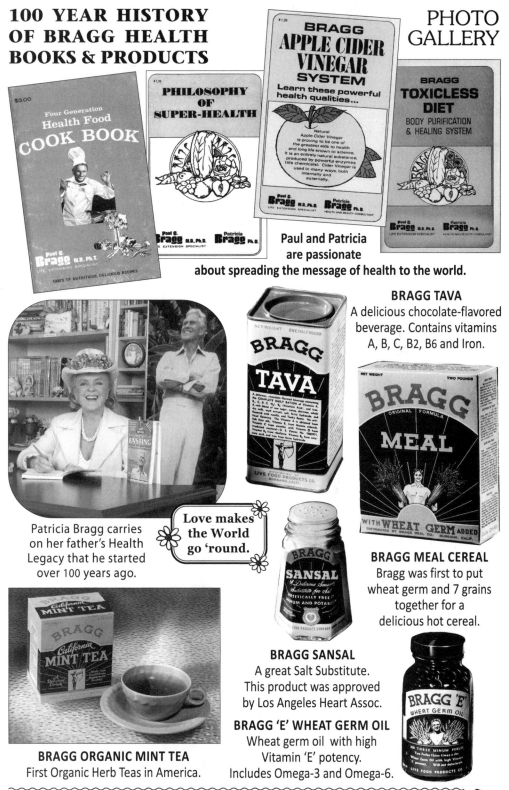

Four Generation Health Food COOK BOOK — $3.00

PHILOSOPHY OF SUPER-HEALTH

$1.25 — BRAGG APPLE CIDER VINEGAR SYSTEM — Learn these powerful health qualities...

Natural Apple Cider Vinegar is proving to be one of the greatest aids to health and long life known to science. It is an entirely natural substance, produced by powerful enzymes (life chemicals). Cider Vinegar is used in many ways, both internally and externally.

BRAGG TOXICLESS DIET — BODY PURIFICATION & HEALING SYSTEM

Paul and Patricia are passionate about spreading the message of health to the world.

Patricia Bragg carries on her father's Health Legacy that he started over 100 years ago.

Love makes the World go 'round.

BRAGG TAVA
A delicious chocolate-flavored beverage. Contains vitamins A, B, C, B2, B6 and Iron.

BRAGG MEAL CEREAL
Bragg was first to put wheat germ and 7 grains together for a delicious hot cereal.

BRAGG MEAL — ORIGINAL FORMULA — WITH WHEAT GERM ADDED

BRAGG SANSAL
A great Salt Substitute. This product was approved by Los Angeles Heart Assoc.

BRAGG 'E' WHEAT GERM OIL
Wheat germ oil with high Vitamin 'E' potency. Includes Omega-3 and Omega-6.

BRAGG ORGANIC MINT TEA
First Organic Herb Teas in America.

BRAGG 'E' WHEAT GERM OIL

"Our lives have completely turned around! Our family is feeling so healthy, we must tell you about it." – Gene & Joan Zollner, parents of 11, Washington

HALL of LEGENDS
Patricia Bragg

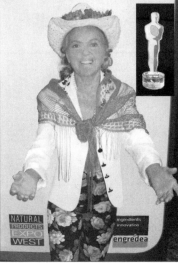

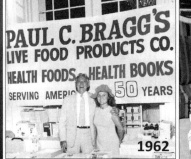

1962

Paul C. Bragg with Patricia, celebrating over 50 years of Bragg Health Products, Books & Crusading worldwide, spreading Health around the world.

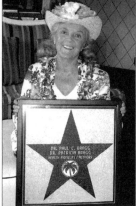

"Palm Spring Walk of Stars" – Patricia with Bragg Star.

Natural Foods Expo in Anaheim with 65,000 attendees from around the world honored Patricia Bragg and her father Paul C. Bragg as treasured Health Food Industry Legends.

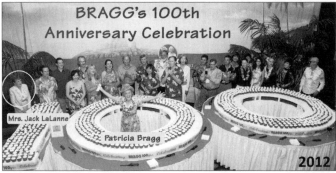

BRAGG's 100th Anniversary Celebration

Mrs. Jack LaLanne

Patricia Bragg

2012

100 Year Anniversary Party celebrated at the Natural Foods Expo in Anaheim

Patricia, Staff & 1,000 Friends celebrated our 100 years of Bragg Healthy Products, Books & Health Crusading! We are proud Pioneers in this Big Health Industry that is helping to keep the world healthier! With Blessings of Health, Peace & Love to You!

Patricia

Bragg Hawaii Exercise Class was founded by Worldwide Health Crusader and Fitness Legend, Dr. Paul C. Bragg. He wanted to create a dynamic, Free Community Exercise Class, and he often taught these classes himself for many years. Patricia Bragg continues her father's health legacy by supporting the Bragg Exercise Class and participates in the class whenever she is in Hawaii.

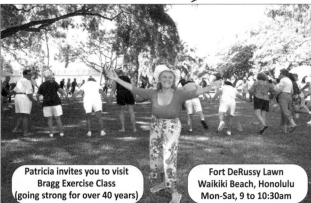

Patricia invites you to visit
Bragg Exercise Class
(going strong for over 40 years)

Fort DeRussy Lawn
Waikiki Beach, Honolulu
Mon-Sat, 9 to 10:30am

"Please make a record of your family history & background. Take pictures – make your own 'Photo Gallery'. Take videos – make movies of your children, spouse, mother and father, family gatherings, etc. These memories are precious & important to save for future generations." – Patricia Bragg

INDEX

A teacher for the day can be a guiding light for a lifetime!
Bragg Books are silent health teachers – never tiring, ready night or
day to help you help yourself to health! Our books are written with
love and a deep desire to guide you to living a healthy lifestyle.
– Patricia Bragg, Health Crusader & Lifestyle Educator

All our dreams can come true – if we have the courage to pursue them.
– Walt Disney

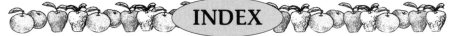

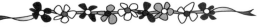

Happiness is a beautiful rainbow in your heart – a real health sparkler!
– Patricia Bragg, Health Crusader & Lifestyle Educator

Dream big, think big, but enjoy the small miracles of everyday life!

Through our actions and deeds, rather than promises,
let us display the essence of love – perfect harmony in motion!
– Philip Glyn, Welsh Poet

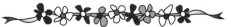

It's the song you sing and the smiles you wear,
that's making the sunshine everywhere. – James Whitcomb Riley

Always do what is right – despite any public opinions.

Please observe and respect the Laws of Mother Nature and God.

What sunshine is to flowers, smiles are to humanity. – Joseph Addison

*A book is a garden, an orchard, a storehouse, a party, a mentor,
a teacher, a guidepost, and a counsellor. – Henry Ward Beecher*

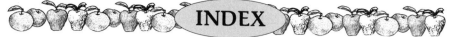

The future belongs to those who believe in the beauty of their dreams.
– Eleanor Roosevelt, U.S. First Lady

Let your inner light happily shine brightly. – Beatrex Quntanna

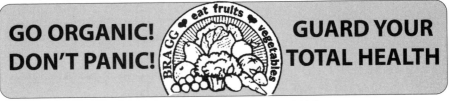

FROM THE AUTHORS

This book was written for You! It can be your passport to a healthy, long, vital life. We in the Alternative Health Therapies join hands in one common objective – promoting a high standard of health for everyone. Healthy nutrition points the way – which is Mother Nature and God's Way. This book teaches you how to work with them, not against them! Health Doctors, therapists, nurses, teachers and caregivers are becoming more dedicated than ever before to keeping their patients healthy and fit. This book was written to emphasize the great needed importance of healthy lifestyle living for health and longevity, close to Mother Nature and God.

Statements in this book are scientific health findings, known facts of physiology and biological therapeutics. Paul C. Bragg practiced natural methods of living for over 80 years with highly beneficial results, knowing that they were safe and of great value. His daughter Patricia lectured and co-authored the Bragg Health Books with him and continues carrying on The Bragg Healthy lifestyle.

Paul C. Bragg and daughter Patricia express their opinions solely as Public Health Educators and Health Crusaders. They offer no cure for disease. Only the body has the ability to cure a person. Experts may disagree with some of the statements made in this book. However, such statements are considered to be factual, based on the long-time experience of dedicated pioneer Health Crusaders Paul C. Bragg and daughter, Patricia Bragg. If you suspect you have a medical problem, please seek qualified health care professionals to help you make the healthiest, wisest and best-informed choices!

Count your blessings daily while you do your 30 to 45 minute brisk walks and exercises with these affirmations – health! strength! youth! vitality! peace! laughter! humility! understanding! forgiveness! joy! and love for eternity! – and soon all these qualities will come flooding and bouncing into your life. With blessings of super health, peace and love to you, our dear friends – our readers. – Patricia Bragg

If I were to name the three most precious resources of life, I would say books, friends and nature; and the greatest of these, at least the most constant and always at hand is Mother Nature and God. – John Burroughs

  Life is a miracle and every day should be treasured, cherished and enjoyed. – Patricia Bragg, Health Crusader

Apple Cider Vinegar - Miracle Health System

BY PAUL C. BRAGG, N.D., PH.D.
and PATRICIA BRAGG

Paul C. Bragg, originator of health stores in America, and world-renowned health crusader Patricia Bragg, introduced America to the life-changing value of Apple Cider Vinegar, with the miracle enzyme known as "the mother." Now a widely popular beverage, this book reveals the legendary health-and life-giving versatility of apple cider vinegar. Following in the footsteps of Hippocrates, who taught the benefits of ACV to his patients in 400 B.C., the Braggs teach dozens of reasons to use vinegar, including as a beauty aid, for skin treatments, in recipes, as an antibiotic, anti-septic, hair-revitalizing rinse, headache reliever, and weight reducer. ACV optimizes digestive health and can reduce or eliminate acid reflux. Paul and Patricia Bragg have helped millions heal and restore their vitality and zest for life through their time-tested understanding of natural health. *Apple Cider Vinegar: Miracle Health System* is informative, entertaining, and invaluable for anyone wanting to feel their best.

Bragg Healthy Lifestyle - Vital Living at Any Age

BY PAUL C. BRAGG, N.D., PH.D.
and PATRICIA BRAGG

Learn the simple strategies of radical health and vibrant wellness that The Bragg Healthy Lifestyle has brought to millions! What is an ageless body? For health pioneers Paul C. Bragg and Patricia Bragg, an ageless body sparkles with vitality, immune strength, mental clarity, and digestive ease. The Braggs teach why a toxic-free diet maximizes energy, supports weight loss, and can help heal illness and disease. In the newly revised *Bragg Healthy Lifestyle: Vital Living At Any Age*, the trailblazing father-daughter team who alerted us nearly a century ago to the dangers of sugar and toxic foods, detail every key aspect of creating and maintaining ageless health, including detoxification, stress-release, nutrition, exercise and the importance of taking charge of not only what goes into our bodies, but practices such as fasting, which release the toxins that may unnecessarily accelerate the aging process. "You are what you eat, drink, breathe, think, say and do," is the Bragg motto. From the foods we eat to our outlook, the environments we live in and even in our physical activities, the authors encourage readers to replace toxins with nutrients, flush out poisons and waste efficiently, exercise, breathe deeply and well, and cultivate happiness and harmony in our daily lives.

Building Powerful Nerve Force & Positive Energy - Reduce Stress, Worry and Anger

BY PAUL C. BRAGG, N.D., PH.D.
and PATRICIA BRAGG

What is Nerve Force and why should you care about it? According to mental health trailblazers Paul C. Bragg and Patricia Bragg, "Nerve Force" is a type of life energy stored in the nerves, muscles, organs, and brain. The more Nerve Force you have, the quicker you can re-charge it, and the healthier, happier, and more satisfying a life you will lead. If you suffer from burnout, stress, fatigue, anxiety, insomnia or depression, this book is for you! We know that the ability to feel joy and peace is essential to a complete experience of vitality and wellness. Our thoughts, our attitudes, our outlook, and our emotional well-being are all dependent on having a powerful "Nerve Force." Just like any muscle that we can develop and strengthen, we can build our Nerve Force so that we are resilient, relaxed, and calm, even during times of stress. Paul C. Bragg and Patricia Bragg show you how with simple mental exercises and suggestions for specific foods that replenish your Nerve Force, as well as foods that deplete it, in this newly revised edition of *Building Powerful Nerve Force & Positive Energy* the father-daughter team explains to readers the reward of paying attention to the energy that is responsible for not only our physical capabilities and our vital body functions, but our ability to process information and feel centered and grounded, no matter what life throws at us. They teach us that maintaining a healthy Nerve Force, leads to a balanced and fruitful life.

Super Power Breathing - For Optimum Health & Healing

BY PAUL C. BRAGG, N.D., PH.D.
and PATRICIA BRAGG

Do you sometimes find that you are panting instead of breathing? Many of us do! This can cause headaches, anxiety, fatigue, and brain fog. The quality of our breath determines the quality of our life! This book teaches us how to breathe in a way that replenishes the body with the oxygen it so deeply craves. "The more effectively we breathe, the more effectively we live," write the authors, world-renowned health pioneers Paul C. Bragg and Patricia Bragg. "Super Power Breathing can make your life-force stronger, calmer and smarter." The Super Power Breathing program has been followed by Olympic athletes and millions of Bragg followers, and is filled with simple exercises for energizing and rejuvenating your breath, and your whole body. Research shows that we use only one-fourth to one-half of our lung capacity with each breath. This starves our body much like if we are depriving it of food. We are slowly robbing our body of its most vital, invisible nourishment – oxygen. In its newly revised form, the Bragg Super Power Breathing Program will give you all the tools you need to shift from shallow breathing to taking deep, oxygen-filled, life-giving breaths!

Authored by America's First Family of Health
Live Longer – Healthier – Stronger Self-Improvement Library

Water - The Shocking Truth

BY PAUL C. BRAGG, N.D., PH.D.
and PATRICIA BRAGG

The water you drink can literally make or break your health. The purity of our water is the most critical element in maintaining radical vitality, and healing from illness and disease. In this newly revised edition of *Water: The Shocking Truth*, health crusaders Paul C. Bragg and Patricia Bragg reveal the dangers of tap water, which research shows can be responsible for many ailments, due to the addition of dangerous chemicals such as fluoride and chlorine. In this book, the trailblazing father-daughter team teach the many functions water performs in the body, from regulating the various systems to flushing the body of waste and toxins. But what if the substance we use to cleanse our bodies is itself polluted? With the mandatory fluoridation of water in the municipal water systems, the authors assert that has been the case for decades. Added to the public water supply to prevent tooth decay starting in the 1950s, fluoride has long been known to be a toxin, used in pesticides and rat poisons. Learn what types of water are optimal to drink, how and why to detox your body with nature's most life-giving liquid, and the health-and-life-saving value of installing a water filter in your shower!

Bragg Back & Foot Fitness Program - Keys to a Pain-Free Back & Strong Healthy Feet

BY PAUL C. BRAGG, N.D., PH.D.
and PATRICIA BRAGG

If you are suffering with back or foot pain, look no further for a comprehensive program that will restore health to the parts of your body that carry you through life! Remember when we were children, and we had the kind of energy and flexibility to play for hours? Agile and active, we could twist, bend, stretch and climb with little effort. However, hours looking at a computer screen, a sedentary lifestyle and poor posture can take their toll. Eventually our backs start to hurt and cramp with every movement, and our feet ache after just a short walk. We start feeling "old." In *Bragg Back & Foot Fitness Program*, the father-daughter team of world-renowned health pioneers, Paul C. Bragg and Patricia Bragg teach how to speed the healing of injuries and develop a strong and flexible back and healthy feet, rejuvenating and re-energizing our bodies in the process. The trailblazing health experts who brought wellness and vitality to millions, including fitness guru Jack LaLanne, outline the keys to a healthy spine, pain-free back and bunion-free feet through nutritional support and clearly illustrated, simple exercises, as well as other tips for posture and massage. Paul and Patricia Bragg reveal the healing properties of herbs, effective ways to practice foot reflexology, how to deal with arthritis, athlete's foot, plantar fasciitis, and foot problems caused by diabetes.

By following the authors' Back and Foot Care Program, you can begin to treat your body as Mother Nature intended you to, and creating painless feet, a strong back and a powerful body will begin!

PATRICIA BRAGG
Health Crusader and "Angel of Health and Healing"

Author, Lecturer, Nutritionist, Health & Lifestyle Educator to World Leaders, Hollywood Stars, Singers, Athletes & Millions.

Patricia is a life-long health advocate and activist, admired internationally for her passionate work promoting healthy living. For many years she traveled the world, teaching The Bragg Healthy Lifestyle for physical, spiritual, emotional health and joy. She was invited to give lectures, visited radio shows, was profiled in magazines and appealed to people of all ages, nationalities and walks-of-life. Together with Paul, she co-authored a collection of ten books, with inspiration and techniques for living a long, vital, happy life. Now in her 90s and living on an organic farm in California, Patricia herself is a testament to these teachings and the sparkling symbol of health, perpetual youth and radiant energy.

PAUL C. BRAGG, N.D., Ph.D.
Life Extension Specialist • World Health Crusader
Lecturer and Advisor to Olympic Athletes, Royalty, Stars & Millions.
Originator of Health Food Stores & Founder of Health Movement Worldwide

Paul C. Bragg was at the forefront of the modern health movement, having inspired generations to turn toward wellness. At a young age, Paul turned his own health around by developing an eating, breathing and exercise program to build strength and vitality. From this life-changing experience, he pledged to dedicate the rest of his life to promoting a healthy lifestyle. He opened one of the country's first health food stores, which eventually led to the creation of the Bragg Live Foods company. With a devoted following, Paul traveled giving lectures and sharing his expertise, while serving as an advisor to athletes and movie stars alike. Even Jack LaLanne, the original television fitness guru, credited Paul with having introduced him to the importance of healthy living. In addition to the books Paul wrote with Patricia, they co-hosted television and radio shows and worked together to bring wellness to the world. Paul himself excelled in athletics, loved the ocean and the outdoors, and radiated with health and a warm smile.

Patricia inspires you to Renew, Rejuvenate and Revitalize your Life with "The Bragg Healthy Lifestyle" Books. Millions have benefitted from these life-changing philosophies with a longer, healthier, happier life!

Take Time for 12 Things

1. Take time to **Work** –
   it is the price of success.
2. Take time to **Think** –
   it is the source of power.
3. Take time to **Play** –
   it is the secret of youth.
4. Take time to **Read** –
   it is the foundation of knowledge.
5. Take time to **Worship** –
   it is the highway of reverence and
   washes the dust of earth from our eyes.
6. Take time to **Help and Enjoy Friends** –
   it is the source of happiness.
7. Take time to **Love and Share** –
   it is the one sacrament of life.
8. Take time to **Dream** –
   it hitches the soul to the stars.
9. Take time to **Laugh** –
   it is the singing that helps life's loads.
10. Take time for **Beauty** –
    it is everywhere in nature.
11. Take time for **Health** –
    it is the true wealth and treasure of life.
12. Take time to **Plan** –
    it is the secret of being able to have time
    for the first 11 things.

YOUR BIRTHRIGHT
HEALTH
CULTIVATE IT

Have an
Apple
Healthy Life!

3 John 2

Teach me thy way, LORD, lead me in a straight path,
because of my oppressors. – Psalm 27:11